"SUCCESS COMES WHEN WE LEARN WHAT TO HOLD ON TO AND WHAT TO LET GO OF."

- HANS SKULSTAD

**Get more mental fitness tips at
www.centerforsportsandmind.com!**

ACKNOWLEDGMENTS

I would like to thank several people who have been invaluable over the several years in developing this content.

I would like to thank all my assistants for their editing and encouragement.

Big thanks to Ellyn Adelmann, Abby Luhrs, Jon Meiers, McKenna Manali, and Judd Ginther.

Most importantly I would like to thank my family – both the Skulstads and Gorres for providing me with the values and inspiration to finish this project.

Most specifically, I need to thank my wife, Jennie, and my son, Hobey, for their support, encouragement, and accommodating my time away. You both inspire me to a better person.

DISCLAIMER

The information presented here should be considered educational and not a substitute for any medical, psychological, legal, financial, or any other professional help.

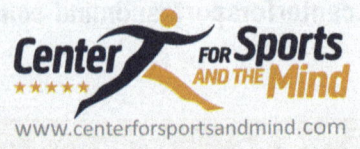

www.centerforsportsandmind.com

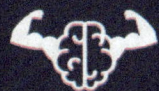 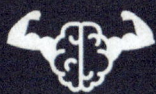

How to Love the Inner Athlete

Q: Becoming a consistently great performer means doing things you have never done before.

These cards require you to do things you have never done before. The concepts presented progressively build on each other. There is a card for each week. If a certain card seems timelier, feel free to use it out of order. The front has mental fitness questions to get you thinking about how to change your Inner Athlete. Be willing to learn. Honestly confront fears. Your awareness will change if you do. Use the provided journal to record your reactions and awareness changes. Increased awareness will help you understand the details needed to be consistently effective.

The following cards require props:
- 17 – deck of cards
- 21 – mouse traps
- 30 – 2 coins
- 32 – calendar and book
- 37 – online numbers grid
- 40 – 2 different color pens
- 41 – straws
- 41 – scissors
- 45 – 4 sheets of paper
- 51 – 6' string with 3 beads or Brock String

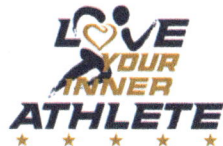

Building mental strength starts with training your thoughts, feelings, and body.

The drills presented here isolate different parts of your Inner Athlete core. Each drill has a purpose that is based on the latest neuroscience and performance research as well as our practical experience. Training your physical core means doing slightly different exercises in the same area. The same is true when training your mental core. Small shifts help to isolate different aspects of mental performance. Some of the exercises are more challenging and uncomfortable even though they are slightly different.

Be open to trying. Pay attention to these things when working through these cards:

1) What distracts you or from the present moment?

2) What emotions, thoughts, and sensations come up in your body? Eventually you may notice a pattern that can help you make needed changes.

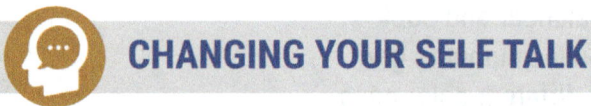

CHANGING YOUR SELF TALK

This section presents effective self talk related to the concept presented. Two methods create the reps needed to make it the "go to" when under pressure. 1) Record the self talk on your phone and listen to it 5–10 minutes every day. 2) Write the new self talk on a daily basis. Write it over and over for 5 minutes or until you fill two sheets of notebook paper. It will be your default self talk when you review it at least 10 minutes at the start and end of each day. Experiment and see what method and times of day work best for you. Keep reviewing the self talk from each week until you can quickly recall it.

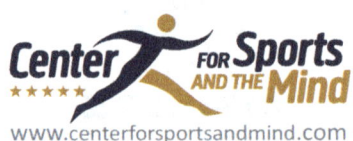

www.centerforsportsandmind.com

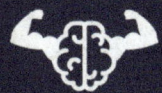 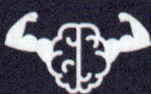
1. Self Scouting – Your Inner Athlete

Q: What's your relationship with your Inner Athlete (your mental game)?

Is it close? Distant? Do you embrace it? Do you fear it? Do you trust it? Do your head, heart, and body work together? Do they fight each other?

There is a power in answering those questions for yourself. It allows you to self scout. Write a scouting report about your Inner Athlete often helps you understand your relationship. Your scouting report needs to include a couple of other things. Identify and write down what's going well.

Second, identify and write down what's missing for your inner athlete. Identify what you need to what would make it more effective and complete. Third, dig deep and identify obstacles that prevent you from making improvements. What do you need to more of, stop doing and start doing.

The scouting report will serve as a map for where you need to go. Keep the report and periodically look back and see how your relationship with your inner athlete grows and changes.

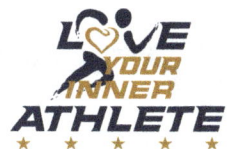

MENTAL ⫴⊢STRENGTH⊣⫴ TRAINING DRILLS

After writing that letter, go through the following steps:

Step 1 – Close your eyes. Form an image of your Inner Athlete. Your Inner Athlete is an alter ego or character you can use to make a shift to your competitive self.

Step 2 – Draw your stomach inward on exhale, allow inhale to arise normally. Repeat 3–4 times.

Step 3 – Picture you and your Inner Athlete as one. Think about the qualities you need to perform. Take notice of the shift it makes in you and think about how you can help each other get the job done no matter whats happening.

Step 4 – Now speed up exhalations (1 per second), do for a minute then take 10 normal breaths. When you are ready, move on to next step.

Step 5 – Encourage your Inner Athlete. Remember your plan to learn more, train it and love it Remember it may take your time to fully realize just who you are.

Repeat this process 3 times (1 min each) and take breaks between each round (10 normal breaths).

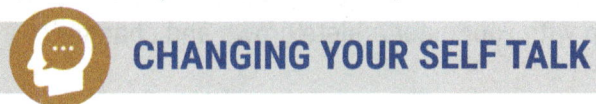

CHANGING YOUR SELF TALK

I train and love my Inner Athlete. My alter ego and inner athlete elevate my performance. When I love my Inner Athlete, I build confidence. I use my Inner Athlete to make adjustments and play hard. I use my Inner Athlete to effectively handles challenges and adversity.

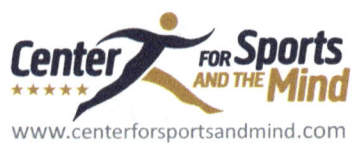

Center FOR Sports AND THE Mind
★ ★ ★ ★ ★
www.centerforsportsandmind.com

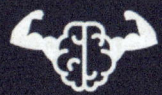 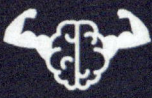
2. Train Your Inner Athlete

Q: Do you know how to train your Inner Athlete?

Many athletes don't or try to do it alone. The training stages below will help you to get clear on the training stages.

Stage 1 – Meet your Inner Athlete. You admit you have things to learn about yourself, your game, and your mental game You don't know what you don't know and understanding what you need to create more consistent performance.

Stage 2 – Get to know your Inner Athlete. You know what to do to improve but you don't change your habits. It's the self–defeating stage. You can't let go of old habits.

Stage 3 – Train your Inner Athlete. You have figured out the "how to" and know what you need to change. Almost there. The consistency skills are there but not automatic.

Stage 4 – Love your Inner Athlete – You got it. You maintain high performance by practicing effective habits. They are part of your daily routine. Accessing the skills of consistent execution are easily accessible.

Moving from one stage to another means there will be times where you feel mixed emotions: feeling uncomfortable vs. comfortable and/or helpless vs. powerful.

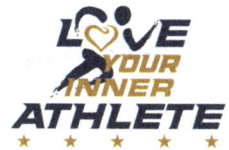

After thinking about the stages, move on to the following drill.

Step 1 – Lie down on your back. Close your eyes and visualize a small flame in your chest. Place your phone or light object on your stomach.

Step 2 – Breathe in through your nose. Notice the intensity of the flame growing as you inhale. Watch your phone rise.

Step 3 – Breathe out through your mouth. Notice the flame diminish. Watch your phone fall.

Step 4 – Use your phone movement to deepen your breath.

Notice how you can control the flame inside you with your breath. Continue for 5–15 minutes.

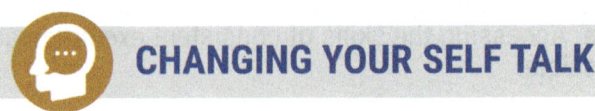

CHANGING YOUR SELF TALK

I accept there are things I don't know about and look forward to learning more. I train my mind every day. I train and work hard even when I don't feel like it. I look forward the struggles and growth that goes with the stages of training.

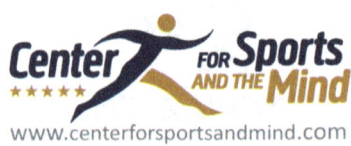

www.centerforsportsandmind.com

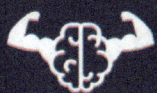 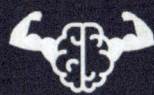
3. Practice Makes Permanent

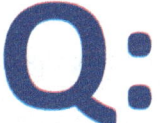 How do you view practice? As something you have to do between games? Or as something you approach with a purpose and goal? What role does practice play in your development?

Viewing practice as an improvement opportunity and a goal for development is key. You need a goal for each practice. Practice makes perfect is a myth.

Practice makes *permanent*.

Having goals and practicing with a purpose helps develop skills; especially through repetition. Skills become hardwired as we repeatedly activate those wires (neurons). "Neurons that wire together, fire together" is a foundational principle of skill and brain development.

To demonstrate how the principle works, try the following: Locate your heart beat. Close your eyes and visualize yourself running sprints or running for 30–45 seconds.

Your heart rate will increase as you activate the same neurons associated with that activity. Practice makes permanent means you can create new habits through purposeful repetition.

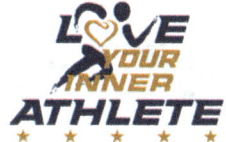

MENTAL ⚡STRENGTH⚡ TRAINING DRILLS

Learn how to calm and relax your body by going through the following steps.

Calm and Relaxed.

Step 1 – Focus on your breathing. Breathe in calm and breathe out tension.

Step 2 – Picture your breath moving through your body.

Step 3 – Picture a part of you that is calm and relaxed.

Step 4 – Repeat silently – "I am becoming calm and relaxed."

Step 5 – With each repetition notice the calm and relaxed feeling.

Continue for 5–10 minutes.

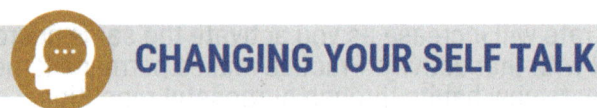

CHANGING YOUR SELF TALK

I have a plan to make new practices permanent. I create new habits through intentional practice. I use repetition to create positive changes. I set at least one goal for every practice.

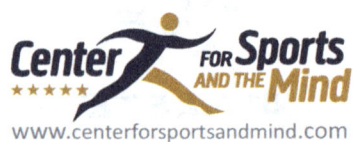

www.centerforsportsandmind.com

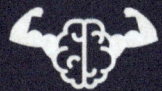 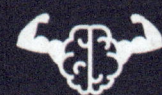
4. The Power of Self Talk

Q: Do you talk to yourself? We all do.

Self talk is the sum of our thoughts and our emotions. It plays a big role in our performance.

When we face adversity, our emotions get kicked into high gear. Self talk kicks in to guide us. How? Automatic self talk takes over. We stop thinking and just do. When the pressure is on, our brain and body go on autopilot, and we can't afford to think. Habits take over.

What does your autopilot say? Training and loving your Inner Athlete can transform you and your performance. It means examining self talk and making needed changes. Learn to change it so it calm your body and emotions. Self talk needs to push, encourage, and action-oriented.

Once you create effective and positive self, you need to strengthen it with repetition. High performance requires effective and encouraging self talk that coordinates your emotions, thoughts, and body.

You are ready to respond instead of react in big moments.

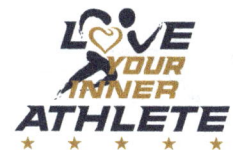

MENTAL ⫴╠STRENGTH╣⫴ TRAINING DRILLS

As you think about your self talk, notice how your self talk, feelings and body work together (or don't).

Progressive Tense and Relax

Step 1 – Focus on your feet. Tense them and then relax them.

Step 2 – Move up your body tensing and relaxing each group.

Step 3 – Tense your entire body and then relax it.

Step 4 – Notice your emotions, thoughts, and body working together.

Repeat 4–6 times with varying speed.

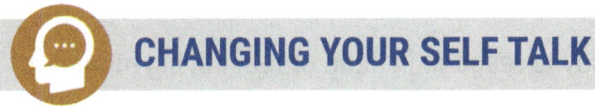

CHANGING YOUR SELF TALK

I look forward to changing my self talk. I perform at a high level because I train my body and mind. I balance and calm my body even under pressure. I perform my best when my thoughts, emotions, and body work together. I use repetition to build strong and effective habits.

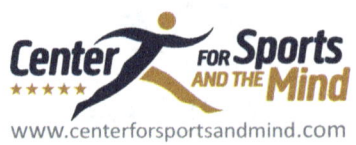

www.centerforsportsandmind.com

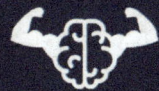 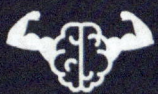
5. "Why" – Love Your Game

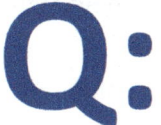 What's Your Why?

Why do you love your game? Why do you love to play? What moments remind you of your love for the game?

When adversity hits, you need to return to your why. It allows you to regain focus and perspective.

This is your WHY.

Step 1 – Identify 3 reasons you love your game and the feelings that you associate with it. Remember these for later.

Step 2 – Identify 3 moments that remind you of those feelings. Pick 3 words that symbolize them.

Step 3 – Use the Quick Coherence Technique of Heart Focus/ Heart Breathing/Heart Feeling Self Calming Skill on the other side of this card.

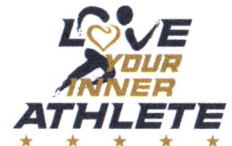

After identifying your why – 3 reasons, 3 moments, and 3 words – go through the following steps.

HEART FOCUS/HEART BREATHING/HEART FEELING: Focus your attention on your heart.

Breathe deeply but normally and visualize your breath going out through your heart. Get into a comfortable rhythm.

Activate your 3 reasons, 3 feelings, and 3 words associated with your love for the game and re-experience them. Expand it to 10 times you felt love, appreciation and gratefulness.

Practice this technique by activating negative experiences and shifting to the positive ones.

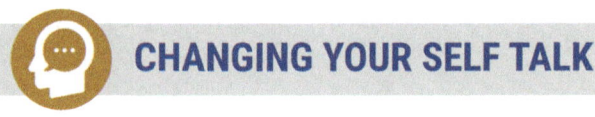 **CHANGING YOUR SELF TALK**

I love my game because (add 3 reasons here). I love feeling (add 3 emotions here). I love moments like (add 3 moments).

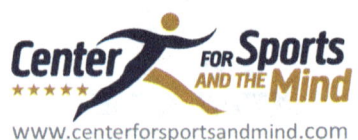

www.centerforsportsandmind.com

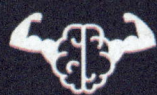 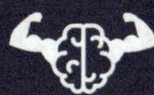
6. Your Default Performance Zone

Q: What's your default performance zone?

Too Tense, Too Relaxed or Flip Flop between the two?

Relaxed	**Optimal Performance Zone**	Tension
Overconfident Disengaged Lack Focus	**The Moment Engaged Balanced Energy**	**Lack Confidence Over Focused Uncontrolled Energy**
Broad Awareness		**Narrow Awareness**

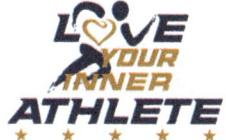

Use the following technique when you need to change your zone: FREEZE, SHIFT, ACTIVATE.

Step 1 – Freeze your thoughts and emotions then step back from them.

Step 2 – Shift your focus to your heart, breathing through the heart with a neutral feeling.

Step 3 – Activate a positive, relaxing, or energizing feeling depending on your default zone. If your default zone is too tense, then activate a relaxing attitude. If it is too relaxed, then activate an energizing attitude. If you tend to flip flop, use the most appropriate for the situation.

Step 4 – Picture your performance from a broad perspective and find an effective attitude or action that will result in you shifting your zone.

Step 5 – Memorize the steps of FREEZE–SHIFT–ACTIVATE. (FSA)

Repeat 3 times. Use this and practice FREEZE–SHIFT–ACTIVATE. Practice it on three stressful situations you are currently experiencing.

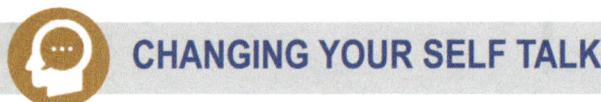

CHANGING YOUR SELF TALK

I use FREEZE–SHIFT–ACTIVATE to return to my OPZ. I engage and let go in my OPZ. I balance my energy by rebooting my brain and focusing on my breath. I focus on the immediate moment. I play with passion in my OPZ. I accept that returning to my OPZ is more important than identifying what took me out.

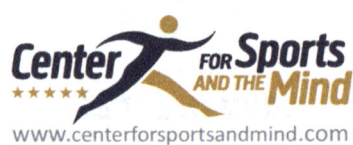

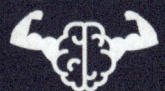 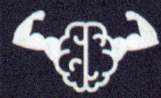
7. The Power of Imagery

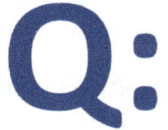 Do you harness the power of imagery?

What's your vision of the future? Imagery is one of the most powerful tools humans use to enhance performance.

Our brains best learn when we use imagery. It ties all of your senses together and activates most of the neural networks in your brain.

Think about a memory you have that's either negative or positive – most often, images and vivid details come up first. We benefit the most when we create an image or scene of the future we want to create.

Our vision of the future is a collection of images we use to envision what will happen and give us motivation.

Try the following exercise on the back of this card to demonstrate the power of imagery. Human nature has a bias toward action. We can use imagery to meet our need for action and move us toward our performance goals.

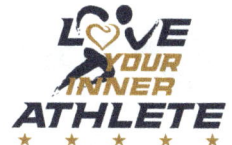

Go through the following steps to see the power of imagery.

Step 1 – Say the first letter of the alphabet out loud and then follow it with the number: A,1, B,2….Z,26. Do this until you get to the end of the alphabet.

Step 2 – On a sheet of paper make a chart with letters in one color and the numbers in another. Try reciting it again and make a mental image in your mind as you do so.

Step 3 – Now try it again without the paper. It will be easier when you use images.

Step 4 – Repeat 4 times.

Step 5 – Visualize the images of what you are doing in the future as you reach your vision and goals. Pair your images with all your senses and emotions.

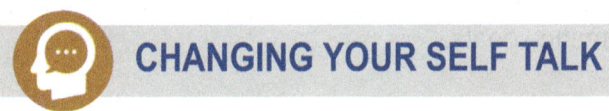

CHANGING YOUR SELF TALK

I use imagery to create consistent performance. I believe imagery is a powerful tool. I use positive imagery and visioning to challenge my future. I know imagery is most effective when I incorporate all my senses.

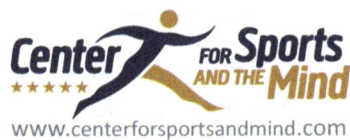

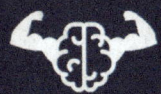 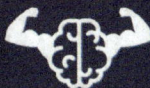
8. Mental Skill – The OPZ

Q: What describes your Optimal Performance Zone (OPZ)?

What 4 times have you have played in it? Identify 4 words that represent you playing in your OPZ.

Relaxed	**Optimal Performance Zone**	Tension
Overconfident Disengaged Lack Focus	**The Moment Engaged Balanced Energy**	Lack Confidence Over Focused Uncontrolled Energy
Broad Awareness		Narrow Awareness

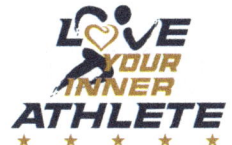

After identifying your 4 words, go through the following steps.

Step 1 – Close your eyes and think of those times. Repeat those 4 words. Recall the sights/sounds/feelings and body sensations of the experience.

Step 2 – Find a spot to your right, left, and center in your field of vision. Stare at each spot for 10 seconds and identify which OPZ performance feels most connected to that spot. This is your OPZ spot.

Step 3 – Alternately tap your legs just above your knees, let your mind go for 1–2 minutes. Stay aware of how your body is feeling.

Step 4 – Check into the good feelings at your OPZ spot. Notice how you feel and let your mind go.

Step 5 – Experience the positive feelings in future performances. Visualize the future performance. Then repeat Steps 1–5 three more times.

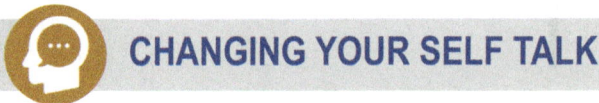

CHANGING YOUR SELF TALK

I play in my OPZ by focusing my four words of _____.

I play in my OPZ by focusing on my OPZ spot.

I play in my OPZ by visualizing my 4 greatest performances.

I see myself playing in my OPZ in future performances.

I love playing in my OPZ.

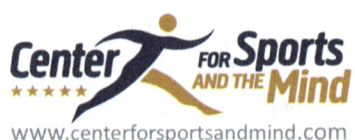

www.centerforsportsandmind.com

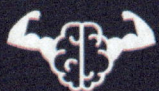 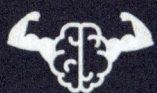
9. Love Your Inner Athlete – Happy Place

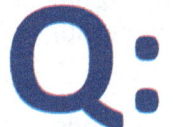 How do you rest, recover, and recharge?

An athlete's life can be crazy and stressful. At times it can feel like there is no safe place or relief from the pressure.

Sometimes you need to go to your happy place. We all have one.

Go there and relax for a minute.

When you do, you love your Inner Athlete. It allows you to rest, recover, and recharge.

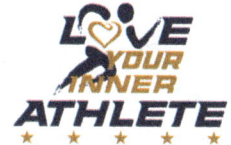

When you need to rest, recover and recharge, go through the following visualization.

Step 1 – Identify a place and time you have felt calm, relaxed, or safe. This may be a place in nature, your room, or a time with friends and family.

Step 2 – Recall all your sensory experiences– sights, sounds, smells, sensations in your body, and tastes. The more details the better. It will make the exercise more effective.

Step 3 – Recall your emotions.

Step 4 – Close your eyes and immerse yourself in that experience while focusing on your breathing.

Step 5 – Tap your legs alternately with your hands for 30 seconds and then rest for 30 seconds. Repeat 3 times.

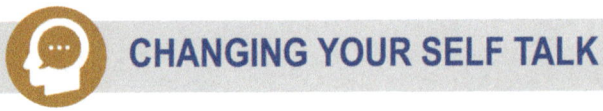

CHANGING YOUR SELF TALK

Going to my happy place allows me to rest and recover. I love recharging in my happy place. It's safe to relax for a few minutes. If life is tense and stressful, it's smart and ok to take care of myself.

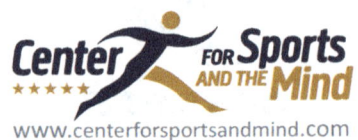

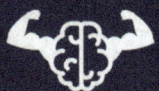 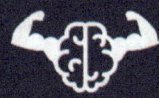
10. Skills – Natural vs Bust

Q: Are you a natural? A bust?

It's important to know if you've been labeled.

Both are fixed mindsets. We encounter them everywhere. Fixed mindsets say we cannot develop new skills and traits. We can change our brains with a mindset shift.

Fixed mindsets help us avoid challenges, fear of embarrassment, and create a false certainty. When you realize that your success depends on effort and as a path to excellence, you adopt belief, faith and trust yourself to find a way to succeed.

The Natural – Believes they are entitled to perform well, and everyone should create perfect conditions. Mistakes are always someone else's fault. Criticism means they are a bust. They trust their physical skills too much and extra effort means they suck. Their default future is a life on easy street.

The Bust – Believes being harshly critical always leads to success. Pointing out mistakes is a punishment and all their fault. They don't trust their physical skills. They think they don't belong. Adversity makes them give up or flip out. Effort is not worth it and means they suck. The default future is a bumpy road filled with landmines and misery.

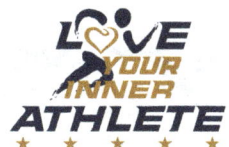

Go through the following steps.

Step 1 – Lie down on your back. Place your phone or light object on your stomach.

Step 2 – Breathe in through your nose. Watch your phone rise.

Step 3 – Breathe out through your mouth. Watch your phone fall

Step 4 – Use your phone movement to deepen your breath.

Repeat for 5–10 minutes.

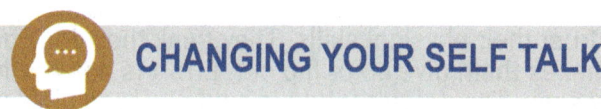

CHANGING YOUR SELF TALK

Mistakes mean I am learning. I refuse the labels of abust or a natural. I learn and improve without being harshly critical. I believe effort = excellence. I believe feedback makes me better. My mind & physical skills help me build a complete game. I believe I can develop my game.

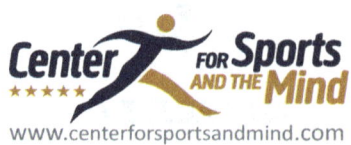

www.centerforsportsandmind.com

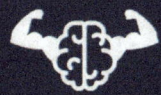 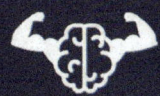
11. Key Knowledge – Attitude

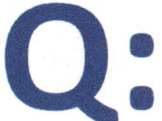 When you have a negative "attitude," what usually creates it?

Someone else's attitude? The situation? Losing? Winning?

Attitudes, just like emotions, can impact our performance. Whether they are energizing or draining, they can be contagious and self–persist.

Attitude and effort are in our control. It can be changed with a conscious decision and effort to shift it. Taking responsibility for your performance means taking responsibility for your attitude and effort.

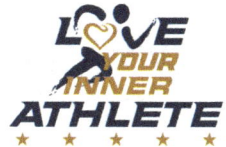

The Attitude Breathing Technique helps you replace draining, negative attitudes with healthier, positive ones.

Step 1 – Recognize Pinpoint a feeling or attitude that is blocking performance. Common blockers are powerlessness, laziness, hopelessness, frustration, anger, or feeling overwhelmed. Identify the body language that goes with each. Make a list of any others that defeat you.

Step 2 – Replace Identify a replacement attitude, then breathe the feeling of the new attitude slowly and casually through your heart area. Do this for a while to anchor the new feeling. Common performance enhancers include energy, poise, intensity, confidence, challenge, fun, and joy. Identify the body language that goes with each. Make a list of those that boost you.

Step 3 – Practice shifting from one attitude to another until you can shift quickly.

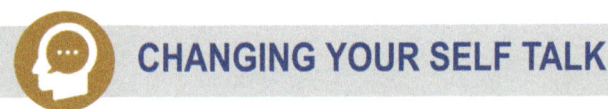 **CHANGING YOUR SELF TALK**

I use attitude breathing technique to choose my attitude. I choose energy, poise, intensity and confidence to transform my performance. I believe taking an optimistic attitude will boost my performance. I am in charge my attitude, effort and energy. I intentionally practice positive body language to maintain a positive mindset.

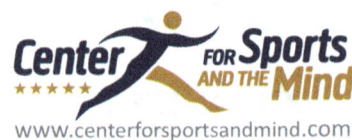

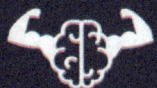 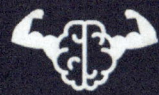
12. Mindset Skill – Self Forgive

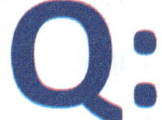 What happens when you make a mistake or fail?

Are you hard on yourself? Do you hold on to the mistakes in hopes of never making them again?

If so, you probably don't know how to self–forgive. Athletes struggle with all of these and the tricky part it that it is usually a combination of all of them.

I CAN'T – you don't know how or what to do.

EMOTIONAL REASONING – your depleting emotions define your view of your play.

I SUCK – acknowledging mistakes means you suck.

THE SPOTLIGHT– everyone will be talking about all your mistakes and how you failed.

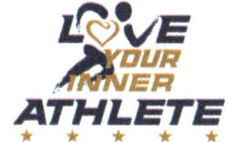

MENTAL ▐⊢STRENGTH⊣▌ TRAINING DRILLS

Think about something you need to forgive yourself for and go through following steps.

Step 1 – Acknowledge a mistake and the emotions it triggers.

Step 2 – Remember it is normal to be disappointed or upset.

Step 3 – Identify what you can learn from the mistake.

Step 4 – Countdown from 200 by 7's and then back up.

Step 5 – Make a conscious decision to forgive yourself.

Step 6 – Focus on the next play & What's Important Now (WIN).

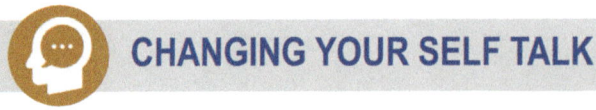

CHANGING YOUR SELF TALK

I accept permission to forgive myself. Forgiving myself boosts my performance. I learn from mistakes without being hard on myself. I forgive myself and so do the important people in my life. Mistakes mean I am learning. Self forgiveness means taking self responsilbility.

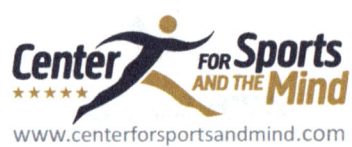

www.centerforsportsandmind.com

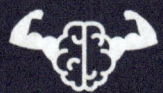 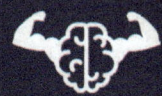
13. Key Knowledge – The Power of Habit

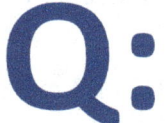 How do you use habits? Do habits run you or do you run your habits?

Understanding habits requires knowledge from Charles Duhigg's *The Power of Habit*.

There are 3 parts to a habit.

1) Trigger – A reminder of something.

2) Routine – Steps we take in response to the trigger.

3) Reward – the payoff we receive from the routine.

We are rarely aware of how this plays out in performance. We often don't question automatic thoughts, feelings, and actions enough because we see others doing the same things. Breaking habits down into small parts give you the framework to change and improve.

Make a list of your habits – the performance killers and the performance boosters. Apply the trigger, routine, reward loop. Performance killers usually protect us from vulnerability and fear – a reward or secondary gain. Performance boosters push us towards vulnerability and fear – overcoming it is the reward.

Habits are hard to stop cold turkey. Its more effective to create a new one. Create new triggers, new routines, and new rewards. Examine all 3 aspects of your habits. You can learn something from the killers and the boosters. Even counting down from 35 by 7's before you complete any step in the loop can modify a habit.

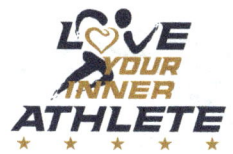

MENTAL ⫞STRENGTH⫞ TRAINING DRILLS

After reflecting on your habit loops, do the next drill.

Recite the alphabet one letter at a time and then say its number in the alphabet. A–1, B–2, C–3, D–4, all the way to Z–26. See how fast you can do it and then do it backwards.

Develop variations like starting in the middle or the 1/3 or ¼ mark add distractions like loud music, sounds or watching TV.

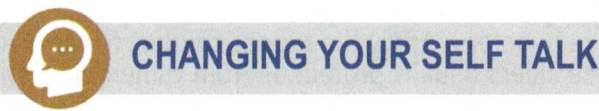 **CHANGING YOUR SELF TALK**

I am aware of my habits. I build performance boosting habits. I change performance killers. I learn new habits. I evaluate my habits and adjust them to make them more effective.

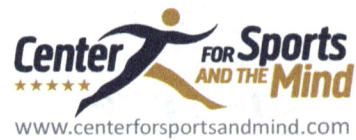

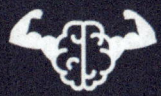 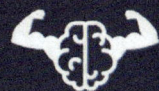
14. The Faith Equation

Q: Do you have faith in yourself?

Do you have faith in the process?

The sum of your faith equation provides you with the belief that you can overcome your areas for growth. What makes up a faith equation? The beliefs you hold about yourself – both positive and negative – and the process.

We often believe that the best way to change is to eliminate the negative beliefs. Building a strong faith equation may seem simple: just be positive all the time. This is impossible.

The key to a strong equation is to have one that is tipped to the positive. It needs some negative. If it is too positive, we get arrogant and feel overconfident. If it is too tipped to the negative, we feel helpless and development stalls.

Development continues when you believe in the process and each side of the equation pushes the other.

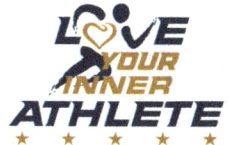

After reflecting on your faith equation, try the next exercise.

Step 1– Sit down and draw your stomach inward on exhales, allow inhale to arise normally. Repeat 3–4 times.

Step 2 – Now speed up exhalations (1 every second), do this for a minute then break (take 10 normal breaths). Repeat cycle 3 times.

Step 3 – Get into a rhythmic flow.

Step 4 – Begin Alternate Nostril Breathing. Close left nostril and exhale through right, inhale through right nostril, do the opposite

Continue up to 20 rounds.

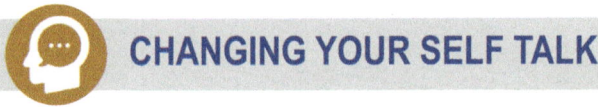

CHANGING YOUR SELF TALK

I keep my faith equation in balance. I believe my strengths and skills allow me to overcome my obstacles. I have faith in myself and the process I use to develop. I emphasize my strengths and remember them when I hit adversity. I see obstacles as temporary problems that can be solved.

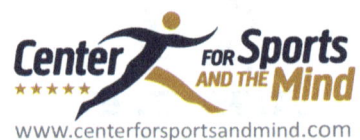

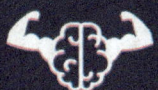 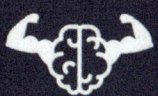
15. Mental Skill – Stress, Your Friend

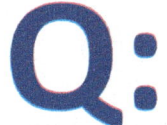 What stresses you out?

School, expectations, not enough time, injuries, nutrition, boyfriend/girlfriend, friends, family, or your future?

What's the best way to deal with it? Avoid it? Pretend it is not there? Approach and deal with it?

Because we associate stress with being uncomfortable we tend to want to do the first two. Those approaches work for a little bit, but it comes back to haunt us in the form of poor performance, meltdown, or freak out. Instead of avoiding or pretending it's not there, we need to face our stress.

Research shows that people who believe that stress helps them experience more success, experience better health, live longer, and feel better.

When we feel stress, we tend to overreact and believe we will be overwhelmed forever. If you make stress your friend, you will get better results. You make stress your friend when you do the exercise on the back of this card.

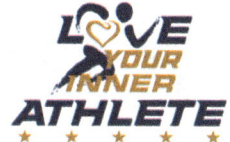

Stress, Your Friend.

Step 1 – Make a written list of the things you need to do.

Step 2 – Read through the items and determine: Priority/ importance, deadlines, and time it will take.

Step 3 – Rank them as A, B, C, in What's Important Now. (WIN).

Step 4 – Focus on the present – Scan your body from head to toe and find 3 abilities you enjoy. You could be grateful that you can see and hear. You might appreciate your ability to plan, and problem solve.

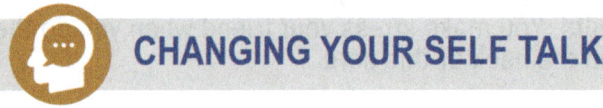

CHANGING YOUR SELF TALK

I can focus, calm and prioritize the things I need to do. I handle stress by focusing on what's important now (WIN). I can contain my stress and there are few problems that are impossible to solve. I have handled stressful situations well before and will again. Seeing stress as helpful promotes growth and development.

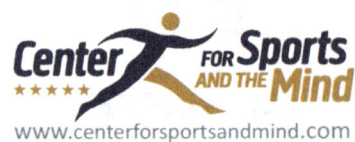

Center FOR Sports AND THE Mind
★ ★ ★ ★ ★
www.centerforsportsandmind.com

9, 10, 11

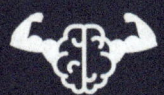 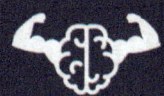
16. Emotional Treadmills – Overthinking

Q: Ever been on an emotional treadmill?

We all have. Overthinking often starts with an emotional event. We can't identify what we are feeling. We try to avoid emotion. Thinking goes into overdrive to identify or avoid.

Emotional perfectionism is the goal. We will feel better if we ignore them. It gets worse. We stop making sense. We know it. Getting off the treadmill means accepting, normalizing, and neutralizing emotion.

Start by making a list of triggers for strong emotions. For each trigger, write down your first thought when triggered. After identifying your first thought ask, "If that thought is true, what's going to happen?" or "What does that mean about me?" Keep asking until you identify at least 20 thoughts for each trigger.

This exercise drills down to what we feel or want to avoid. Most people find common themes and loops. Be mindful that both positive and negative emotions can trigger the treadmills.

Joy and fear can both lead to strong emotions. Don't be afraid. Move toward them and you will move toward better performance.

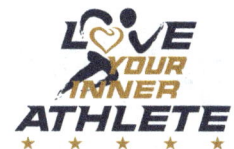

The Celly

Step 1 – Put your palms together. Feel the warmth between them.

Step 2 – Inhale and open your arms like you are celebrating a big play.

Step 3 – Hold your position and breath for count of two.

Step 4 – Exhale slowly and count to 4 as you bring your palms back together.

Continue for 5–10 minutes.

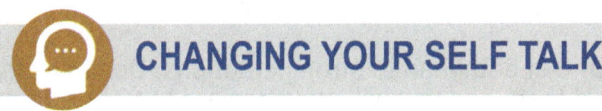

CHANGING YOUR SELF TALK

I accept that emotions are a part of sports and life. I can feel strong emotions and perform. My play improves when I stay off emotional treadmills. Treadmills lead me to nowhere. With time, effort, and patience, I learn what runs my emotional treadmills.

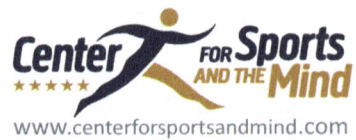

www.centerforsportsandmind.com

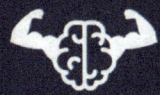 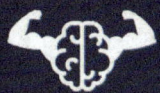

17. Mental Skill – Tryouts

Q: There is no denying they are a stressful. How stressful are tryouts for you?

You're being evaluated. You are exposed. The pressure builds. Everyone is watching. Here are some important things to remember as you prepare for tryouts.

1) The Wow – Don't give into the temptation to push for the "wow." Evaluators know how to look for the details. Such as being in the right position, effort, and consistency.

2) The Controllable – Your effort, attitude, body language, and play are in your control. Don't try to play to what you think everyone is looking for. What makes a great player is different for everyone. If you try to please everyone, you please no one. Including yourself. Play true to yourself and your game.

3) Trust Your preparation – A tryout is a moment in time. It's not career defining. Take the plays that come. Make confident decisions.

4) Avoid the Draft – Although it's tempting, don't draft the team in your head as you play. It takes your focus off your play. It creates the illusion of certainty. Find ways to relax, be intense, and stay poised.

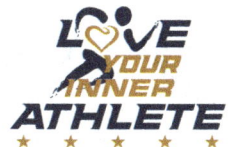

After thinking about your approach to tryouts, try the following exercise.

Step 1 – Sit 15 feet away from a calendar at eye level.

Step 2 – Hold a deck of cards face down about 10 inches from your face and level with belly button. Flip the first card over, focus on which suit it is.

Step 3 – Drop the card and shift focus to the date at the bottom right of the calendar. Flip the next card over and focus on it. Repeat the process until all the cards are gone.

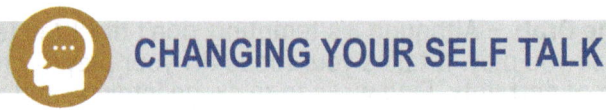

CHANGING YOUR SELF TALK

I focus on my play and my game during tryouts. I trust my preparation. I perform through uncertainty. I avoid the draft game.

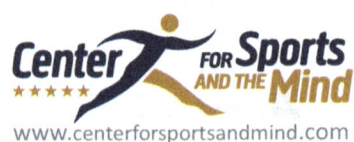

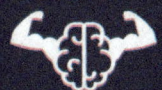 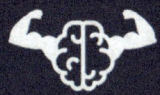
18. Self Scouting – The Discount

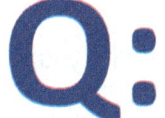 When do you discount or minimize yourself?

Is it in your preparation? Is it after a performance?

Many athletes discount the positive even when they get the results they desired. Many athletes have "go to" and hidden beliefs that keep them from building resilient confidence.

They usually come in the form of "yeah, buts". What's your favorite?

- I made a mistake on _____.

- I got lucky on_____.

- It wasn't perfect.

The "yeah, but" before these statements changes their meaning. Athletes often think this is a way to protect them from the expectations of success. They don't want to appear arrogant.

Using "yeah, buts" keeps you stuck in the mediocre middle and out of the high performing zone. Breaking into the high-performance zone creates stress. You change and leave your old self behind.

You will welcome a confident and resilient Inner Athlete when you stop discounting your confidence and accept that you can be great without being perfect.

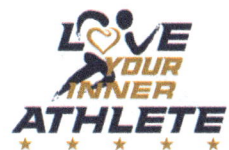

Focus on positive experiences that build confidence and do following exercise.

Square Breathing

Imagine as you breathe that you are making a square with your breath. Each intake & expulsion describes a side, each equal. Keep your rate of breath normal, but equal on each in-breath and out-breath.

Box up your old self and embrace the new.

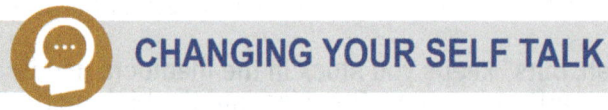

CHANGING YOUR SELF TALK

I handle increasing expectations from success. I build a confident and resilient Inner Athlete. I refuse to discount my play. I handle my changing self and changing performances. I put the "yeah, buts" aside and handle expectations of myself.

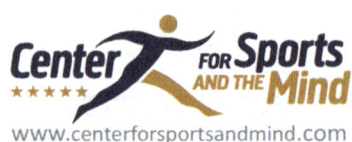

www.centerforsportsandmind.com

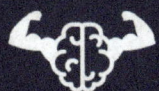 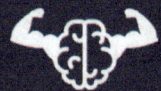
19. Obstacle Mind Traps

Q: What's your most often used mind trap?

Adversity = bad – Adversity should be avoided.

Performance defines me – Play well, you and the world are good. Play bad, you and the world are bad.

Pressure of expectations – You play to please everyone watching.

Constant self judgment – You judge your play every moment.

Over focus on mistakes – You only notice mistakes and ignore success. These mind traps keep us circling in our emotions.

These particular traps shift your attention away from the moment.

What triggers you to get stuck in mind traps? Identify 3 triggers. Being aware of them and what triggers will help keep you out of the traps.

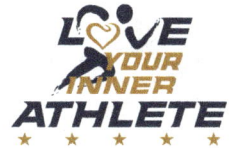

Use the following exercise with each trigger and mind trap.

Step 1 – Close your eyes and try to focus on 1 of the following 3 things: sounds around you, your breathing, or sensations in your toes.

Step 2 – Open your eyes and find a sign, logo, or anything with words. Read it and spell it 3 times.

Step 3 – Scan your environment for sounds.

Step 4 – Scan your environment for smells.

Step 5 – Focus on your breath and the sensations it creates in your nostrils or stomach. Try to notice everything about this one breath.

Step 6 – Focus your attention on the sensations in your toes. This forces your mind to sweep through your body.

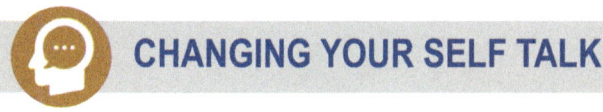

💬 CHANGING YOUR SELF TALK

I shift my focus by scanning for sounds, smells, my breath, or the sensations in my toes. I shift my focus by finding a sign and spelling out the words 3 times. I am aware of my mind traps and redirect them to an external focus.

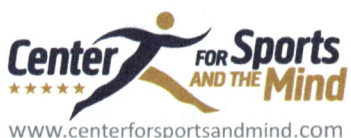

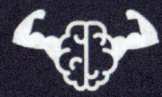 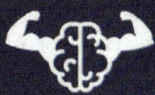
20. Mental Skill – When Your Body Talks

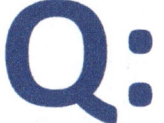 What does your body say? Body language.

Does your body do all your talking? Is it hard for you to hide your emotions?

Coaches, scouts, and teammates all notice body language. It gets noticed most when it reflects frustration, tension, defeat, and a lack of confidence.

When you sense those emotions, you can change how your body talks. You can change them to something positive by changing your body.

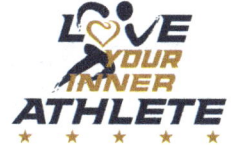

Start with neutral body language and do the following steps.

Step 1 – Take an easy deep breath. Stand up – shake up your body.

Step 2 – Widen your stance – plant your feet. Being big = confidence.

Step 3 – Reach for the ceiling. Now the walls on either side.

Step 4 – Drop your arms to your sides. Roll your shoulders up and back.

Step 5 – Pinch your shoulder blades together like you are holding an ice cube on your spine.

Step 6 – INFLATE. Take up as much space as possible. Puff up – be big but don't get out of control.

Repeat 5 times.

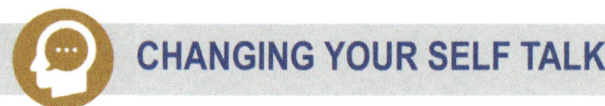

CHANGING YOUR SELF TALK

I am aware of my body language. I change my body talk with the INFLATE exercise. I transform my body by calming my emotions. I learn to manage my body talk by spending time and effort on it. Being frustrated is a part of sports, but I use the frustration to energize me.

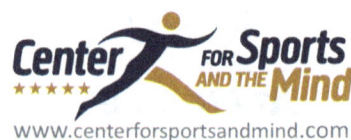

www.centerforsportsandmind.com

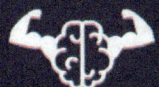 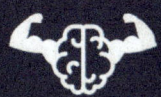
21. The Container

Q: Ever feel like you keep making the same mistakes? Ever wonder why?

It may be because we can't set aside poor past performances. What past performances do you need to put away but not completely forget?

This exercise will help you identify them and contain them. When you are ready, you can take them out to learn from them and forgive yourself.

Step 1 – Close your eyes and take a deep breath. Slowly alternately tap your legs above knees.

Step 2 – Visualize yourself sweeping all stressful events you have experienced. You will see a collective pile and nothing specific.

Step 3 – Visualize a container or dumpster big enough to hold the pile. Take note of color, size, and where it sits.

Step 4 – Visualize your pile moving into the container or dumpster.

Step 5 – Add a valve on top to add new things at other times. Add a valve on the side to take 1 thing out at a time to talk about with a trusted person. Add a sign that says, "Open only when it serves to restore, recharge, or rejuvenate me."

Step 6 – Repeat until most of the pile is in the container. Take note of the experiences and write them down.

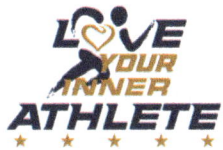

After finishing the container, do this exercise.

- Set a mouse trap.

- Set it again with your eyes closed.

- Activate the mouse trap with your palm and hold hammer with fingers.

Do all these until your fear decreases and you get comfortable with these steps. This process is the process of becoming comfortable with the uncomfortable and working through your fear.

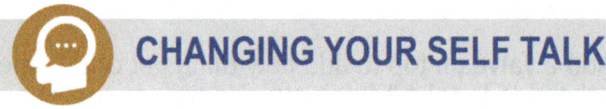

CHANGING YOUR SELF TALK

I use my dumpster to set aside stressful events. I set aside my past performances. I identify and overcome my traps. I overcome fear by facing it.

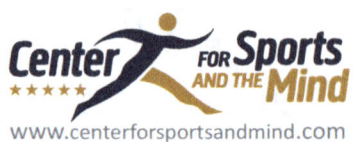

www.centerforsportsandmind.com

14

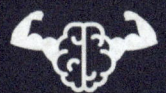 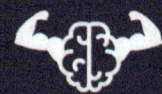
22. Compliance vs Commitment

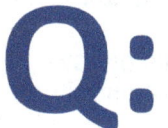 What are you committed to?

Being committed to your game and your Inner Athlete requires more than just complying with what is expected of you.

Some coaches and athletes ask themselves to comply with process. Compliance looks different than commitment. Compliance deceives by leading to short term success. Compliance means you punish yourself for failures.

Athletes who use it as their primary method of motivation say, "I have to…..", and then complain about how hard it is.

Their play lacks emotion, creativity, passion, and fun. When you train and play with commitment, your performance changes. You play with resilience and determination.

Commitment means you are in it for the long haul. Short–term results, setbacks, and losses are just a part of the process. You are willing to play hard and take risks.

You commit to challenging your future to get the most out of yourself.

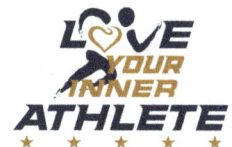

MENTAL ⫽⊢STRENGTH⊣⫽ TRAINING DRILLS

Step 1 – Sit down and close your eyes.

Step 2 – For 5 minutes visualize your life as if you are watching it as a movie. Focus on as many positive aspects as you can.

Step 3 – Think about commitments you need to make or have made. Imagine your future self and succeeding in keeping those commitments to yourself.

Step 4 – Then write a story about what you did to keep those commitments. Make a list of all the things happened.

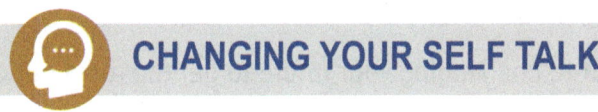 **CHANGING YOUR SELF TALK**

I commit to my Inner Athlete. I look forward to doing the work it takes to move to the next level. I commit to playing with poise, intensity, creativity, and passion. I commit to enjoying the process.

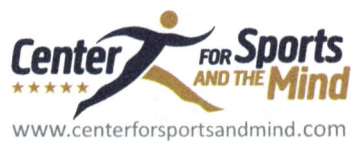

www.centerforsportsandmind.com

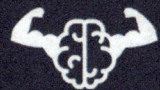 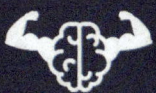
23. Self Scouting Skills – "I Can't"

Q: What have you been told you can't do?

Negative messages subtly come from our culture, ourselves, and the people around us.

"I can't" statements suggest that change is not likely to occur. It says you will not learn and is a self–limiting belief. They create blocks and glass ceilings leading us to see these as signs we cannot improve. Sometimes it means we are afraid to push through them.

Step 1 – Write down negative messages you have consistently heard from others about you. Try to identify at least 4.

Step 2 – Identify experiences that disprove the statement. Look for many as you can no matter how small.

Step 3 – Whenever you find yourself repeating negative messages, redirect yourself to a sign near you to reboot the brain. Then remind yourself of the things you have done to counter those beliefs.

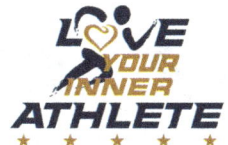

After thinking about those experiences go through the following steps.

- Find a sign near you and read it.

- Spell it out letter by letter.

- Spell it backward.

- Read it again.

- Repeat 3x with 3 different signs.

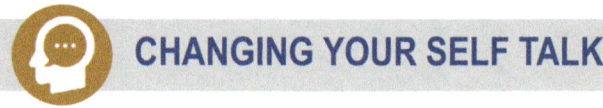

CHANGING YOUR SELF TALK

I overcome and reframe negative messages. I have strengths that make me an effective performer. I encourage myself when things are difficult. I motivate myself with optimism. I overcome my fears.

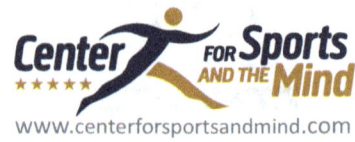

www.centerforsportsandmind.com

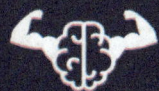 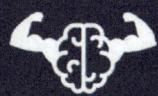

24. Mindset Skills – Failure = Learning

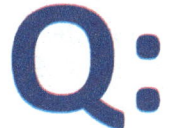 How do you view failure?

Many athletes believe that failing indicates lack of skill. Sometimes coaches and athletes view failures as defining.

Identify which myths about failure keep you stuck in a fixed mindset.

Failure Myth – Failing means I am a failure.

Superhero Myth – I am not good unless I am number one and the best.

Perfection Myth – I can achieve "perfect."

Never Myth – I'll be this way forever and never get it.

—

Step 1 – Identify – skills you struggled with but mastered.

Step 2 – Remind – yourself that you can have learned many times.

Step 3 – Change – expectations. Be You not a Superhero.

Step 4 – Progress – can be achieved but perfection cannot.

Step 5 – Reboot – get all your brain online.

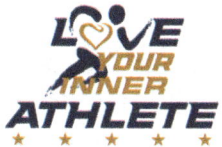

After thinking about those myths go through the following steps.

Palm/Fist Squeezes – Alternate squeezing fists for 1 minute.

Alternate pressure with thumb on opposite palm for 1 minute.

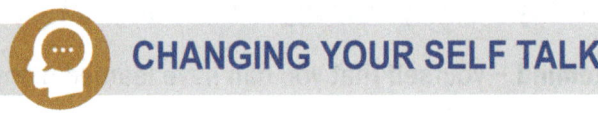

CHANGING YOUR SELF TALK

I stay gritty in the face of failing. I play my game and am an effective performer. I progress and grow my game. Perfection is a myth. I can change and develop with effort and patience. I take responsibility for my attitude and effort as a result of my performance.

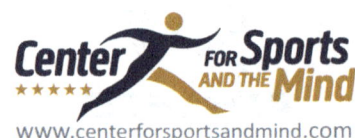

www.centerforsportsandmind.com

4, 5, 6

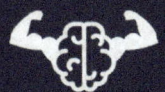 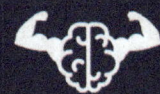
25. Key Knowledge – Fear vs Danger

Q: Is there a difference between fear and danger?

Our fight, flight, freeze responses protect us from danger.

Humans today face far fewer life threatening situations than we did hundreds of years ago. The explosion and speed of information that is present today often misleads us to believe that there is no difference.

When we confuse them, we overreact, and drama ensues. The panic monster shows up. Sports can be dangerous but most of the time they are not.

Our brains are designed to provide us safety, survival, and significance. Fear is a normal part of sports. Training your brain to distinguish between the two comes with the 3p's – **perspective, preparation, and practice.**

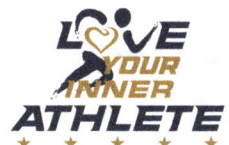

Step 1 – Preparation – Remember you are prepared for these moments. Your preparation allows you to see fear as just fear.

Step 2 – Perspective – Concentrate on how your feet feel on the ground. Imagine breathing through your legs, this can help ground the body and stop the panic monster.

Step 3 – Practice – Your 3-Part Breath. Take a normal breathe then exhale in 3 parts (inhale, exhale–pause, exhale–pause, exhale–pause, inhale). That is 1 rep. After 10 reps, lengthen the exhalation naturally, easily, and without strain.

Continue for 5–10 minutes.

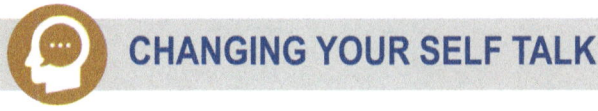

CHANGING YOUR SELF TALK

I know the difference between fear and danger. I push through fear without drama. I use my preparation, perspective, and practice to face my fear.

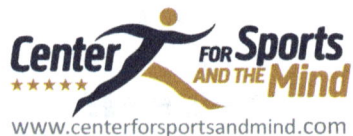

www.centerforsportsandmind.com

11, 16

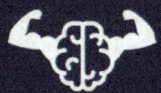 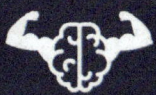

26. Key Knowledge – Slumps

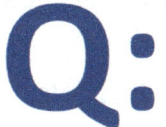 Ever been in a slump? They suck. Really suck.

The slump monster shows up. No one is immune.

Consistency is replaced by helplessness and fear. Things are not going to change ever. We press. We guess for "the cause." The magic bullet. The ONE thing. "If I can just find 'the answer,' relief, life will resume as usual."

These are the guidelines for busting a slump:

1) Consult with coaches to see if there is a problem with your fundamentals or a physical problem.

2) Practice patience – stay focused.

3) Trust your skills and abilities. Don't give into the temptation to overhaul things.

4) Stay optimistic. Nothing is permanent.

5) Stop guessing. Focus on what's important now. There is no "the answer." There are many reasons that create slumps. We can't see them all. With patience and time, solutions emerge.

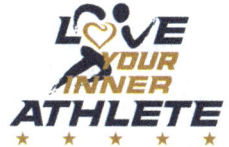

Think about slump you have experienced and do the following exercise.

Step 1 – Visualize your breath relaxing your core and moving down your body. All the way to your toes and up to your head.

Step 2 – Picture a power or cause greater than you – God, fate, the earth, or whatever works for you.

Step 3 – Imagine the power lifting responsibility off you.

Step 4 – Visually watch it leave your shoulders and prepare to learn from the process. Follow the slump busting guideline.

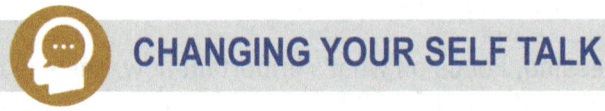

CHANGING YOUR SELF TALK

For 5 minutes repeat these sentences: I beat slumps. I practice patience when the slump monster shows up. I use my resources to help me correct fundamentals. I accept that there is no one answer or solution. I trust myself and ability to change my performance.

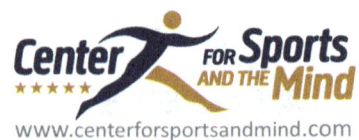

www.centerforsportsandmind.com

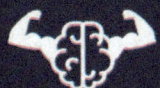 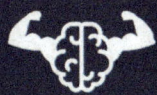
27. Mind Traps – Avoid the Slides

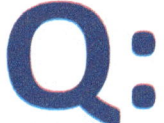 What makes you slide down an emotional valley?

What gets you started on emotional treadmills to nowhere?

When something happens that challenges the plan and creates difficult emotions, it can be tempting to hit a slide. The deeper the slide, the more work it takes to climb back out.

Knowing the steps makes it easier for you to stop them and limit their negative impact.

S – I Suck – You believe that everything about you sucks.

L – Loser – You are a "loser" and a failure with a miserable future.

I – Isolation and Imagine – You isolate and imagine the worst including being alone forever.

D – Downer – You let everyone know you are down. People try to pick you up, but you resist and stubbornly stay down.

E – Escape – The pain feels unbearable and inescapable. Poor decisions result. You turn to drugs, alcohol, food, or anger to make it go away. You make impulsive decisions. You damage relationships.

Deep slides can be prevented by not getting to the 'I' in 'SLIDE'. Remind yourself that your mistakes don't define you. You have solved problems in the past. People care about you. You are successful.

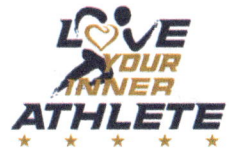

MENTAL ⫼STRENGTH⫼ TRAINING DRILLS

After thinking about what your slides, do the following exercise.

Step 1 – Focus on your breathing. Breathe in calm and out tension.

Step 2 – Picture your breath moving through your body.

Step 3 – Picture a part of you deep inside that is calm and relaxed.

Step 4 – Begin repeating silently – "I am becoming calm and relaxed."

Step 5 – Each time you will feel that part that's calm and relaxed.

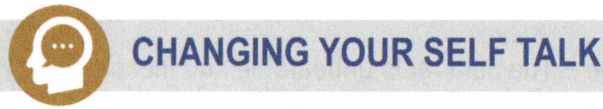 **CHANGING YOUR SELF TALK**

I avoid deep slides. I connect with others when I face disappointments and strong emotions. I acknowledge difficult emotions and let them pass.

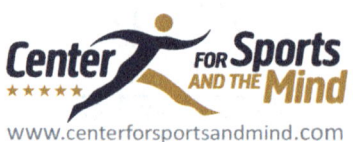

www.centerforsportsandmind.com

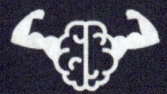 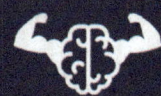
28. Good to Great – The Fear of Success

Q: Are you afraid of success? It happens. It's a human reaction. What scares you about success? The expectations, the pressure, or being in the fishbowl?

Success requires leaving the mediocre middle. Moving from good to great requires doing things differently. When we move into the high performing zone, things happen that may want to make us go back to the mediocre middle.

1) We lose the company of others and feel alone.

2) We are targets of the members of the mediocre middle.

3) We fear falling back to the middle. If we were to fall, we would get embarrassed for all to see.

All 3 create fear, expectations, and pressure. So, when you get there, what do you do?

Remind yourself you put in the work and trusted the process to create your success. It was not an accident. Tell yourself the same hard work plus a little more will help you maintain your place. Ignore the crowd, and accept you do things different. Focus on the joy you feel as you experience success.

Remember you are not really alone. Enjoy and look forward to the challenge of other pushing you for your spot.

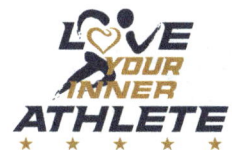

MENTAL ⫩STRENGTH⫩ TRAINING DRILLS

Step 1 – Locate the spot just below your pinky. Tap on it.

Step 2 – Close your eyes for 5 taps and open for 5 taps.

Step 3 – Without moving, look down and left for 5 taps.

Step 4 – Circle your eyes in a complete circle while tapping.

Step 5 – Reverse the circle. Then count to 5 aloud while tapping.

Step 6 – Hum 5 varied notes while tapping. Count to 5 aloud again.

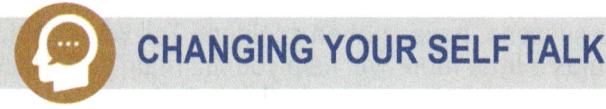

CHANGING YOUR SELF TALK

I handle success because I do the work to get there. My success is built by trusting and following my process. I maintain success by putting in more work and finding new challenges. Being and doing things different builds my success. I look forward to challenge of maintaining my success.

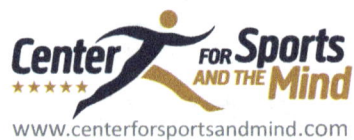

www.centerforsportsandmind.com

1, 18

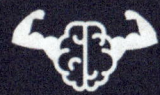 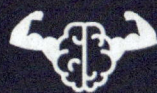
29. Self Scouting – "I Never"

Q: What are your "I never's?"

Finish this sentence at least 5 different ways.

"I never_____".

Try to exhaust all things that come to mind. Think about all parts of your life. We engage in these statements to protect us from responsibility for our performance.

Using "I never" may be a sign that you are using a limited measure to evaluate reality. The second step in your process is to ask yourself what your "I never's" are when the difficult events happen.

Try the exercise when the following happens:

* When I get rattled or upset, I never......

* When things don't happen, they way they should, I never.....

* When I screw up, I never......

* When I get criticized or attacked, I never.....

* When others screw up, I never......

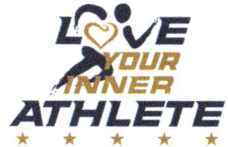

After thinking about your "I never's", do the following exercise.

Step 1 – Sweep through your body from head to toe and find 3 abilities you approve. You could be grateful that you are breathing, blinking, or moving.

Step 2 – Breathe in through your nose and out through your mouth.

Step 3 – Breathe in thinking energy and breathe out thinking tension.

Step 4 – Repeat until you find 5 things you can be grateful right now.

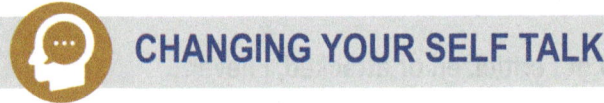
CHANGING YOUR SELF TALK

I evaluate with my performance without using all or nothing terms. When I get rattled I let the feelings pass. When unexpected things happen, I view as a chance to push beyond my limits. I show my gratefulness for the things I have by playing hard. I listen to my own voice and believe I do things that are out of my comfort zone. I believe I can have faith and trust in myself and abilities.

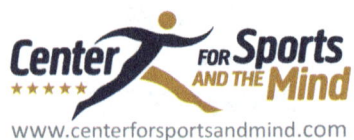

www.centerforsportsandmind.com

11, 15

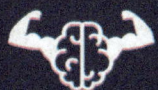 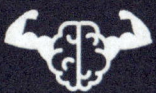
30. "I Hope" – Superstitions

Q: What are your superstitions? What are your hopes?

We often confuse the two.

We see our hopes as long off dreams we don't have the power to reach. We leave our hopes to chance by relying on superstitions. Sometimes we leave our performance to chance.

When we hope but take no action, our hopes become something that we may or may not ever get to. Instead of figuring out how to make them a reality, we wait for something to happen.

Many athletes try to create that "something" with luck and superstition. What superstitions and good luck charms do you need? When we cling to superstitions, we take ourselves out of our performance equation and give up control to the illusion of control.

Instead of relying on the good luck charms and superstitions you need to make something happen, get energized and do the work. Use your emotions, your faith in yourself and your great past performances to fuel this change.

Remind yourself that you have been the something that changes. Identify the superstitions you need to let go of and stop using it.

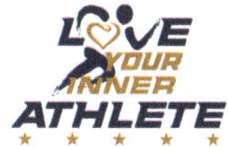

After examining your superstitions, do the following exercise.

Step 1 – Place 2 coins an inch apart with the face side up.

Step 2 – Position your head directly above the coins with your nose pointing directly in the middle of the coins (about 16 inches above them).

1. Cross eyes to make the 2 coins appear to be 3.

2. Concentrate on the coin in the middle, hold for a count of 10, and release.

3. Count to 10 again as a break and then repeat the process 5 more times.

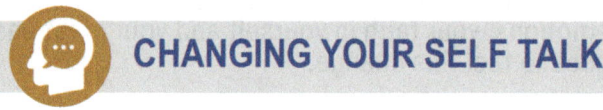

CHANGING YOUR SELF TALK

I rely on my ability and minimize superstitions. I control my performance. I look forward to using my faith in myself, my emotions, and reminders of great performances to make things happen. I accept that I am responsible for my own performance.

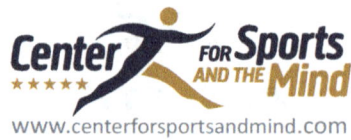

www.centerforsportsandmind.com

12, 15

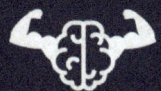 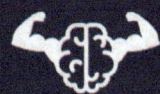
31. Brutal Realities

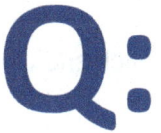 What are your brutal realities?

These are the obstacles we wish away and don't want to be there. The things we may want to hide.

Many times, athletes work to remove the emotions that our brutal realities create. This often results in avoidance.

Instead, you need to take a problem–solving approach. We can often identify brutal realities by looking at performances we do not feel good about.

What 3 past performances have been the most difficult to forgive, forget and move on from?

Recall thoughts about yourself or your performance. The emotions you felt, what you saw, heard, smelled, and tasted. Notice any patterns that emerge – the opponent, the circumstances, and common triggers for performance.

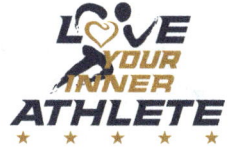

After thinking about those experiences go through the following steps.

Step 1 – Find a focal point and focus on it.

Step 2 – Without moving your head, move your eyes back and forth for 1 minute.

Step 3 – Find a focal point far away and then find a focal point close to you. Move your eyes back and forth from near to far for 1 minute.

Repeat 3 times.

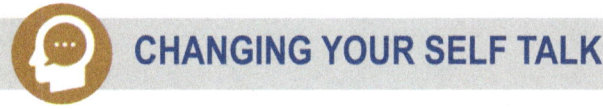

CHANGING YOUR SELF TALK

I define myself and my future. My past performances do not define me. I can play in the here and now. I can use eye exercises to calm myself. I forgive myself and learn from my past performances. I look forward to problem solving the obstacles I face.

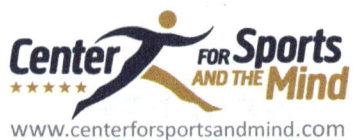

www.centerforsportsandmind.com

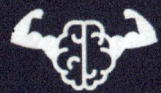 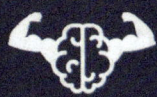
32. Mental Skill – Goal Setting

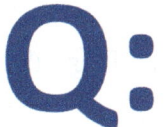 What are your goals?

Setting goals is more than just writing down stats that you want to put up.

Some things keep us from meeting them –the game plan, the opponent, or the role we are asked to play. Statistics are outcome goals.

Consistent athletes make process goals. These are things you have the power to change. An example might be – Your relationship with your inner athlete. Develop the characteristics of the high performing mindset – challenging yourself. Competing with your last performance. Being able to self–forgive. Seeing failures as learning. Being comfortable with being uncomfortable.

Step 1 – List the characteristics, mental skills, and sports skills you need to develop to be consistent.

Step 2 – Rate yourself from 1 to 8 on that list. Have a trusted coach rate you as well.

Step 3 – List daily habits and goals that develop your inner athlete.

Step 4 – Set weekly and monthly goals.

Step 5 – Make a spreadsheet with columns for daily, weekly, monthly and long term. Add a 5th column labeled benefits and list the way your life will change if you meet your goals. You can download ours at centerforsportsandmind.com/resources.

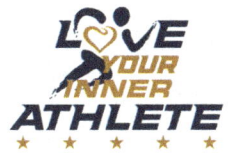

After completing your goal setting, do the following exercise.

Step 1 – Put a calendar on the wall and grab a book. Move 15 feet away.

Step 2 – Read a line from the book and then look up and read the calendar.

Step 3 – Do this for 5 minutes.

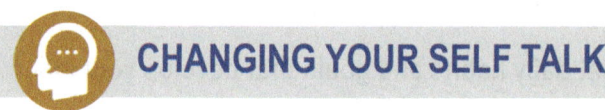

CHANGING YOUR SELF TALK

I set process goals to develop consistency. I set process goals that help me develop my inner athlete. My goals keep me focused on process and daily habits for success. I check my progress toward my goals once every two weeks.

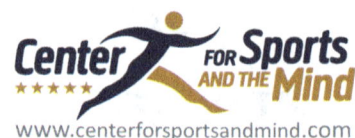

www.centerforsportsandmind.com

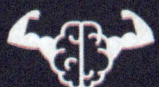 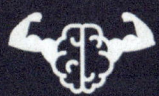
33. Comfortable with Uncomfortable

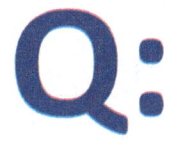 Do you get out of your comfort zone?

Developing your skills requires you to move into the uncomfortable. The best performers learn how to be comfortable with being uncomfortable.

Why? Your opponents game plan to make you uncomfortable. Which one of the 3 "F's" are you most likely to do when uncomfortable?

Fight (Aggressive) – Flight (Shut Down) – Freeze (Paralyzed)

When you are uncomfortable remember you can be comfortable with uncomfortable by remembering:

Preparation – Rely on what got you here. Practice.

Perspective – It's a moment and not life threatening.

What You Know – Focus on what's true and accurate.

It's Normal – Growth requires the uncomfortable.

What's Important Now – Focus on it.

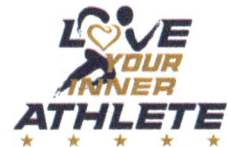

After reflecting on the how to get comfortable with the uncomfortable, do the following exercise.

Step 1 – Find a corner in the room.

Step 2 – Imagine a wire connecting a point to your nose.

Step 3 – Picture an object on the wire.

Step 4 – Slide the object down and back to the point.

Step 5 – Alternate between point and nose for 30 seconds.

Repeat 4–5 times.

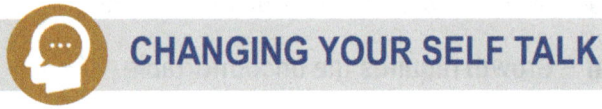

CHANGING YOUR SELF TALK

I focus on what I know to be true. I stay composed under pressure and the uncomfortable. I stay focused on the moment. I look forward to getting comfortable with the uncomfortable. I trust my preparation why I am uncomfortable. I maintain perspective when uncomfortable. I accept the uncomfortable is part of sports and life.

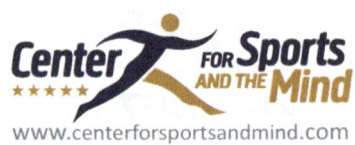

www.centerforsportsandmind.com

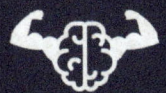 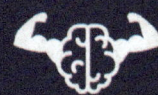
34. Momentum – Real or Fake?

Q: What do you do when the opponent has the momentum? What do you do when you or your team has it?

It is viewed as an athlete's superpower. It's real. We can feel it and know it's there even if we cannot touch or see it. It can propel us to victory or resign us to defeat.

What's most important is how you respond to it. It can be deceptive. Leading us to believe that the outcome is determined. It sabotages effort. Stemming momentum requires emotional energy and effort. Maintaining it requires the same.

It's important to respond instead of just react. Responding means you continue to execute your game plan and make necessary adjustments. Reacting means you panic and abandon what got you there.

When you give in to negative emotion you play with fear and believe that momentum is against you.

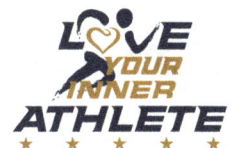

After reflecting, follow the steps in this exercise.

Step 1 – Identify times you have felt momentum.

Step 2 – Play out those moments in your mind.

Step 3 – Notice the energy and emotions it creates.

Step 4 – Identify times you have lost momentum.

Step 5 – Shift between the 2 – alternating between extremes.

Step 6 – Project a movie of each on the wall. Notice how you respond and shift.

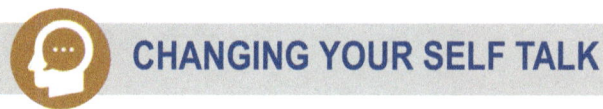

CHANGING YOUR SELF TALK

I look forward to responding to changes in momentum. I use energy and effort to maintain or change momentum. My role and job stays the same no matter what momentum says.

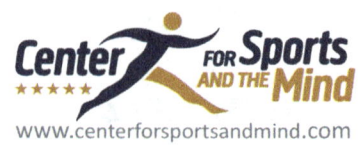

www.centerforsportsandmind.com

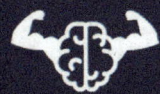 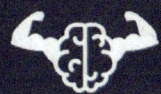
35. Self Scouting – "I Wish"

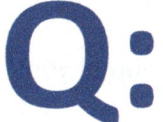 If you had 3 wishes for your Inner Athlete, what would they be?

For your athletic skills? For your life? Write them down. Review them. Notice any themes?

Wishes reflect the things we want to happen but do not think we have the power to make happen. Wishes might be things we believe we have no control over. A belief that we are not good enough. Refusing to accept the reality of what is happening now.

Ask yourself how this applies to your wishes. With some focused thought you might be able to see there is something you can do to make your wish into a goal.

You may find a way to stop wishing and focus on what you have the power to change.

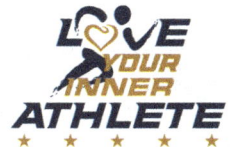

After thinking about those experiences go through the following steps. Do this activity with your head still – just eye movements. If you struggle, start with head and eye. Read aloud and follow the instructions.

Breathe in, look straight ahead – Breathe out, look to top of your head

Breathe in, look straight ahead – Breathe out, look to your right ear

Breathe in, look straight ahead – Breathe out, look to your left ear

Breathe in, look straight ahead – Breathe out, look down to your chin

Breathe in, look straight ahead – Breathe out, look down to your right

Breathe in, look straight ahead – Breathe out, look down to your left

Breathe in, look straight ahead – Breathe out, look up to your right

Breathe in, look straight ahead – Breathe out, look up to your left

NOW, JUST BREATHE!

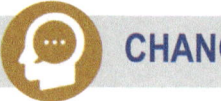 ## CHANGING YOUR SELF TALK

I work to achieve my goals. I focus on what I can control. I stretch myself to reach for hard to attain goals. I can make the most of what I have learned, earned, and developed. Being satisfied with what I have done so far does not mean I stop working. I consistently look for ways to get better. I know I can take action to change my physical and mental game.

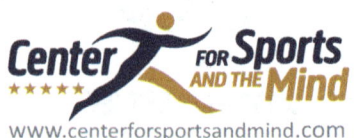
www.centerforsportsandmind.com

15, 20

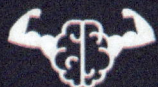 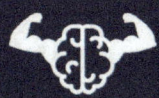

36. Mindset Skills – Plan and Adapt

Q: Can you coach yourself?

Planning and adapting requires self coaching.

It means knowing what to do when you are off. Knowing throughout the season and in the moment.

Great athletes learn how to plan, problem solve, and adapt. Our great coaches often can be used as a resource to help us plan, problem solve and adapt our performance.

The difference between great performances and poor performances is self coaching.

Step 1 – Identify great coaches who have raised your game.

Step 2 – Identify 4 qualities that made them great for you.

Step 3 – Identify 4 things you learned from them.

Step 4 – Identify 4 things they said that made you better.

Step 5 – Identify 4 moments they coached you well and the emotions you felt.

Use these to coach yourself and plan, problem solve, and adapt.

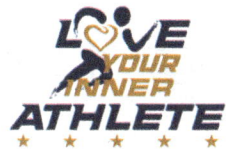

After thinking about your great coaches, go through the following steps.

Find a focal point that is far away. Then look at your nose. Move back and forth for a few repetitions. Think about the times they have coached you well.

Remind yourself of the 4 qualities, things you learned, things they said, and the moments they coached you well. Then pick from each category and create an internal power coach.

Then with each word move your focal point from near to far. i.e., smart,– look far – Relax look near.

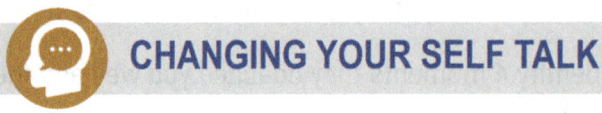

CHANGING YOUR SELF TALK

Good preparation allows me to perform my best. I adapt during competition and the season. I have the courage to identify problems in performance and make changes. I use my past power coaches as a resource for changing my performance. I draw on my power coaches to self coach.

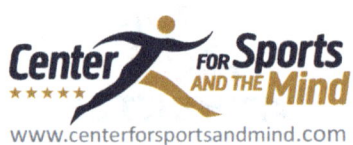

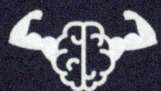 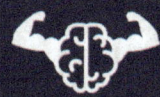
37. Mental Skill – Own the Moment

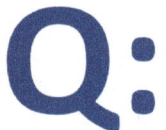 What triggers you to leave the present moment?

Athletes often mentally slip out of the now and into the future or the past. You can train present moment focus.

Use the 45 second drill.

When drifting – Stop – make a commitment to focus for 45 seconds. After it's over, notice how your energy and focus changed. Try this with any activity. Try this with a numbers grid.

Go to www.centerforsportsandmind.com/resources to find a grid to practice. Start the stopwatch on your phone.

Step 1 – Circle the numbers in order – 1,2,3…. up to 100.

Step 2 – See how long it takes you to finish.

Step 3 – Create variations – 60 seconds, 10#s in the middle of 100 –add music, loud sounds, the TV, try it in a crowded room – Try to lower your elapsed time each time.

Step 4 – Get into a routine of doing them at least 3x/week.

Step 5 – Notice your thoughts, emotions, and body. What distracts, calms and refocuses you?

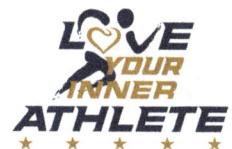

After trying the moment drill, do the following exercise.

Recite the alphabet one number at a time and then say its letter in the alphabet. 1–A, 2–B, 3–C, 4–D, all the way to 26–Z.

See how fast you can do it and then do it backwards.

Develop variations like starting at different points, add distractions or do every other set in the sequence.

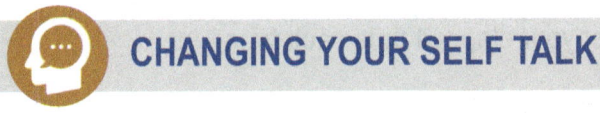

CHANGING YOUR SELF TALK

I get great results when I pay attention to my learning and training cycle. Routines and habits help me develop present moment focus. Present moment focus is something I can practice. When I drift, I can refocus with the 45 second drill.

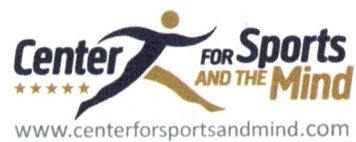

www.centerforsportsandmind.com

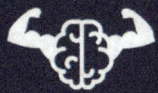 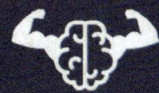
38. Self-Scouting – "I Should"

Q: How often do you say "I should really _____"?

We often tell ourselves we "should" do something. When you start with "I should" it is a fear of commitment or a lack of it. It means "I don't feel like it."

The moment "you feel like it" never arrives. When we do not do the things we know we need to, it breeds more "should".

It may be a sense of obligation or burn out. It may look too big. It may not be enjoyable.

Break whatever it is into small steps and find some part of it you can enjoy. Commit and find the energy to focus on what is in your control – your love of the game, your why, and your joy of meeting your goals.

Accept and confirm your commitment to do the hard things even when you could be doing something else that is more fun.

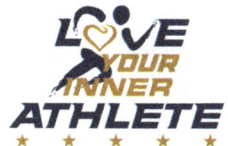

After identifying what you need to commit to, do the following exercise.

Look at a wall 10 feet away.

Step 1 – Move eyes in a zig-zag pattern from the top left corner of the ceiling, tracing the top edge of the wall to the right corner in a straight line, and then down diagonally back to the left (only 2 feet below the starting point).

Step 2 – Stop when you hit the bottom right corner of the wall. Reverse and do it again.

Step 3 – Find a spot on the wall that represents 12 o'clock.

Step 4 – Slowly move eyes around clock 3 times. Stop 2 seconds at 12.

Step 5 – Start at 6 and do the same counterclockwise and then do once more but start at 12.

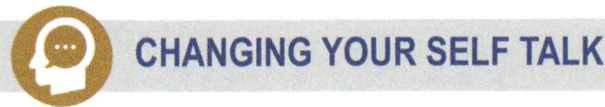

CHANGING YOUR SELF TALK

I generate energy and determination to do the things I don't enjoy. Great performances require me to do difficult things. I look at difficult things as an opportunity to make myself better. I find things to look forward to even when it may not be fun.

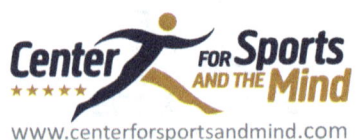

www.centerforsportsandmind.com

12, 15, 18

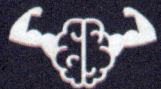 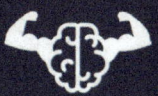
39. Love Your Inner Athlete – Your Team

Q: Who has your back? Who can you trust? To support and love you? To tell you to change? To tell you the truth?

We all need people to bring meaning and purpose to our lives. We need human contact when times are tough or when we are struggling.

Sometimes we need to recall those people and what they mean to us because they are not immediately available or because they are no longer with us.

Make a list of 4 or 5 people who you respect and trust and who will support, encourage and challenge you.

Make a list of qualities they have that make them support people for you. Make of list of emotions that you feel when you think of them.

Put the list on your phone's notes and look at it every day.

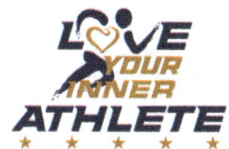

After reflecting on your team, try to the following breathing exercise.

Breathe in for a count of 5, hold for 2 and out for 7.

Repeat breathing in calm, breathing out tension with each inhale and exhale. While maintaining that pace think about someone who has taken care of and protected you.

Visualize in as much detail as you can. Then think about the qualities that make them good caretakers.

When ready, think about times they have taken care of and protected you. Feel the emotions that go with them taking care of and protecting you.

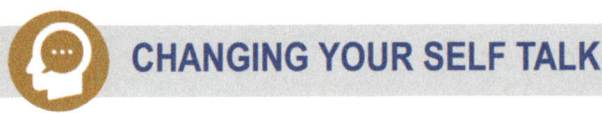

CHANGING YOUR SELF TALK

I have the courage to use my support team when help is needed. It is normal to ask for help from my support team. I can trust my support team to be honest, encouraging, supportive, and give me feedback. I connect with my support team. Connecting with my team calms and energizes me.

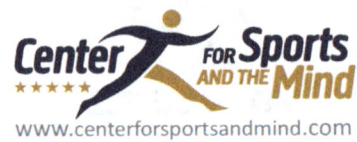

www.centerforsportsandmind.com

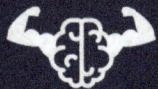 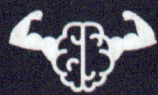
40. Self-Scouting – "I Always"

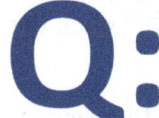 Sometimes we give into the temptation to generalize our experiences.

"I always" is a often used phrase.

Finish this sentence in at least 3 different ways. "I always____"

Try to exhaust all things that come to mind. It can be about any part of your life or any time . Write them down. These messages often come from our culture, experiences, performance and ourselves.

What you say and believe about yourself is important. Always statements suggest that there is no exceptions. You have no control over what choices you make and how you respond. It may also mean you have an inaccurate view of how you respond.

There may be exceptions to statements like "I always work hard."

There is a benefit to finding times you don't so you can do more.

See if you can find exceptions to your "always"... Look and see if there is one thing you can change to break the pattern of what happens to you.

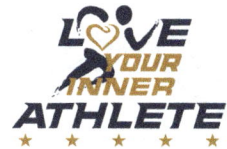

After reflecting on the "one thing" you can change, do the following self calming and vision exercises.

Eye Jumps – Hold 2 different colored pens in front of you and move your eyes back and forth; change the distance between the pens, depth and height "eye jumps" Repeat 3x's.

Dueling Pens – Call out the color of one pen, to draw the eyes to it. Then move the other pen and draw the eyes to the new pen. Look at the tip of each pen and fixate on it with your eyes. Then call out a pen color again, and so on. Repeat 3x's. Then alternate but call out the color opposite of the one you are looking.

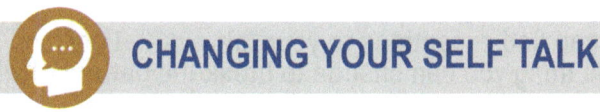

CHANGING YOUR SELF TALK

I correct mistakes in my performances. I believe that I change my performance. Things change and nothing lasts forever. I give myself permission to challenge my future by changing one thing in in my habits. I perform in any circumstances.

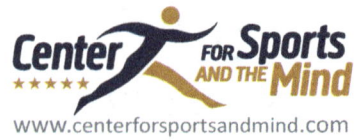

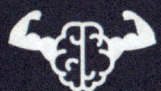 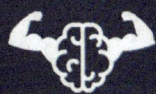

41. Challenge/Compete with Yourself

Q: How do you challenge yourself?

Do you do different or uncomfortable things?

Challenging yourself means you put yourself in situations that make you uncomfortable.

Too often we compare ourselves to others which distracts our focus from our performance. Growing your game means you take risks and fail.

It is easy to stay good. Going from good to great requires challenging yourself to be better than your last performance.

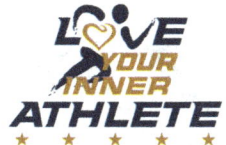

Challenge yourself with the following exercise.

This straw breathing technique will challenge you to learn the 6 breaths exercise and activate your relaxation response.

Step 1 – Cut a straw in half and hold it in your fingers.

Step 2 – Inhale normally and naturally through your nose. Your lips and face should be relaxed.

Step 3 – Exhale fully through a plastic drinking straw – make sure you have exhaled all the air out of your lungs.

Step 4 – Repeat this exercise for 5 minutes. Challenge yourself by trying to take only 6 breaths/minute or 30 total.

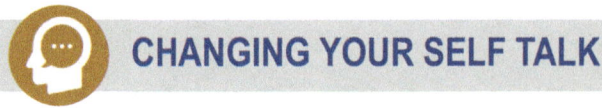

CHANGING YOUR SELF TALK

I can challenge myself with the 6 breaths exercise. Using the 6 breathes exercise activates my relaxation response. My relaxation response will enhance my performance. I challenge myself to be better than my last performance.

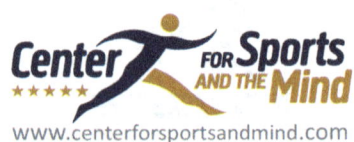

www.centerforsportsandmind.com

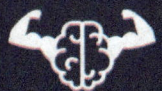 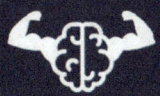
42. Mental Skill – Centering

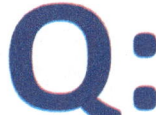 What throws you off balance? What brings you back?

Staying centered requires a strong mental core.

As long as we are breathing there is more right with us than wrong with us. The people who care about us recognize the same. These are the people who love us for who we are not what we are.

The following exercise is designed to help you find the people who center you. You can use them and a centering breath together to bring you back to center.

Step 1 – Make a list of 25 people who care about you and then add 25 more.

Step 2 – Identify 3 general reasons they care.

Step 3 – Identify the ones who stop caring if you fail at your sport and any that love you for that instead of who you are.

Step 4 – Identify 4 positive emotions about the 50 people.

Step 5 – Connect with some of them in person or by imagery to center yourself.

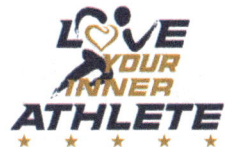

MENTAL ⫘STRENGTH⫘ TRAINING DRILLS

Challenge yourself to center yourself with the 4 emotions exercise.

While feeling those 4 emotions:

- Take a breath in for the count of 5.

- Hold for the count of 2.

- Breathe out for the count of 7.

- Repeat as needed.

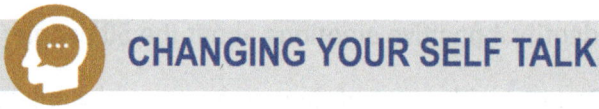

CHANGING YOUR SELF TALK

I effectively use a centering breath. I center myself by remembering who loves and cares for me for who I am. I center myself by remembering the 4 centering emotions of the people who love me.

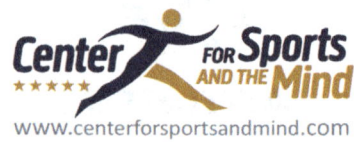

www.centerforsportsandmind.com

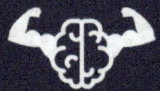 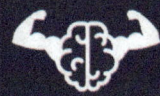
43. The Contagious Teammate

Q: Are you that person? The contagious one.

Which "that person" are you? The basher, the builder, or the settler?

The basher is negative, moody, and hard to be around. The builder is positive, encouraging, and fun to be around. The settler accepts mediocrity and is fine with whatever happens.

All are contagious.

What do builders do? Own their emotions – recognize them and treat them like gas. It will pass. They intentionally let them pass. Everyone can.

As an example, think of a time you were in a funk, and you ran into an old friend who brings you joy. That time and memory pulls you out. You make an automatic and quick change to your emotions.

Everyone can be a contagious emotional game changer who can make others feel positive, energetic and confident.

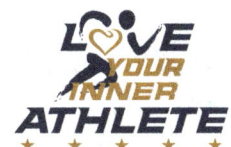

Reflect on which contagious teammate are you.

Step 1 – Observe yourself and everyone around you from a 3rd person lens. Pay attention to their body language, emotion, and energy.

Step 2 – Notice the vibe in the crowd or in your team.

Step 3 – Give yourself 45 seconds to identify and experience what you see, hear, feel, smell, and taste.

Step 4 – Make a shift to a poised, relaxed, and confident feel.

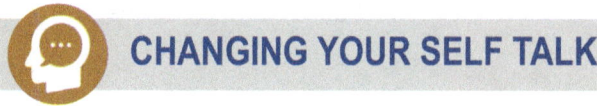

CHANGING YOUR SELF TALK

I own my emotions and take responsibility for them. I give myself permission to feel emotions and let them pass. I lead by being contagiously positive, energetic, and confident. I recognize uncomfortable emotions and become contagiously positive. I infect my team with energy, poise, and confidence.

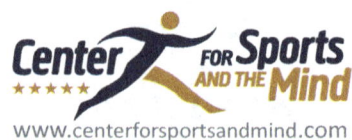

www.centerforsportsandmind.com

4, 5

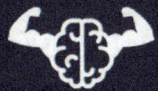 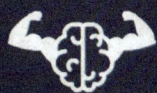
44. Self-Scouting – "I Know"

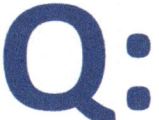 When you get feedback, how often do you say, "I know"?

You may be closing the door on possibility. It is code for "Shut up!!!!"

Don't be afraid to admit that you don't know. Many athletes fear that admitting not knowing means they are dumb or don't care.

To change your performance, you must learn more about yourself and the process of change. It means being open to feedback.

Chasing new knowledge. Asking questions. Digging in and embracing curiosity. Read something that will do all the above.

Talk and learns from watching others who execute more effectively or are more skilled. Don't be afraid of what you don't know. Every athlete's performance is influenced by things they don't know, and the most effective ones are open to discovering what that may be.

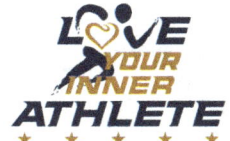

After accepting there are things you don't know, do the following exercise.

Step 1 – Sit down on a chair, cushion, or mat.

Step 2 – Take a full, easy inhalation through your nose.

Step 3 – As you exhale, sound the numbers "o-n-e", "twoooo", and "threeeee" separately for 5 seconds each – breath in and out normally between each number.

Step 4 – Keep repeating step 3, gradually increasing the length of the exhalation sounds until you reach 15–20 seconds each.

Step 5 – Do this exercise for 5–10 minutes.

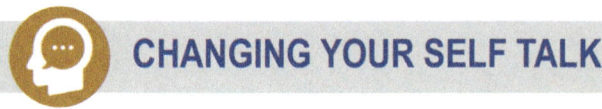

CHANGING YOUR SELF TALK

I accept the fact that I may not always know what I need to do to improve. I accept feedback and challenges as opportunities to improve. I actively accept coaching. I learn from others who strive for excellence.

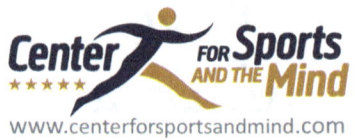

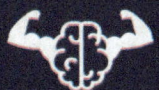 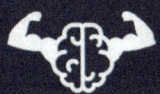
45. Mental Skills – Attention

Q: What distracts you?

What keeps you from maintaining your attention on the present moment?

Many athletes excel because they can quickly shift their attention. Some athletes can achieve laser focus while others struggle to maintain attention. Others have trouble making transitions from one thing to another.

Practicing these exercises will help you improve your attention skills.

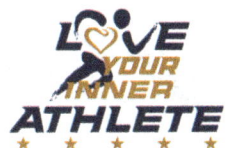

The Memory Game.

Get a deck of cards. Distribute them face down and create a grid of cards that is 7 by 7. You will have a few extra cards that will create and incomplete row. Play the memory game.

Start a stopwatch. Start by turning over 2 cards at each turn. As you create matches set the matched cards aside and continue until you get all the matches. Record your time. Each day you do this try improve your time.

To add difficulty, add distractions – loud music or noise, people talking, randomly removing some cards. Notice how you handle the pressure, frustration, and distractions and the strategies you use to shift.

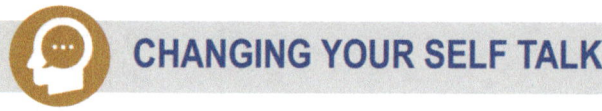

CHANGING YOUR SELF TALK

I shift my attention based on the needs of the situation. I shift my attention when I need to. I transition from one activity to another.

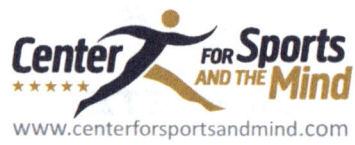

www.centerforsportsandmind.com

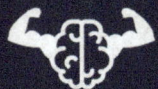 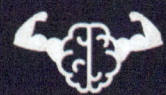
46. Mental Skill – Smile

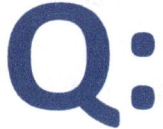 What makes you smile?

Put a smile on your face right now.

What did you think about? What did you feel?

Now think about a person or a time you dislike. The smile left your face, didn't it? Now smile again.

Don't under any circumstances let it go. Try thinking about that person. You cannot maintain that negative emotion as long you are smiling.

Notice it takes less energy and effort to be positive versus negative.

Identify at least 5 people whose presence brings a smile to your face and gives you a feeling of joy and love. Next, identify at least 5 times one of those people made you laugh and smile.

Now identify 5 times you have made someone else smile. Now think of 5 things you feel gratitude for.

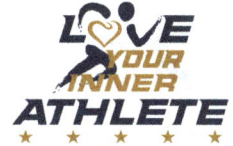

MENTAL ⅃⊢STRENGTH⊣⅃ TRAINING DRILLS

Try the following exercise.

Close your eyes and visualize the 5 people who bring a smile to your face. Notice how you feel and think. Every detail. Your breathing.

Now visualize the times that make you laugh and smile. Notice how you feel and think. Every detail. Your breathing.

Now visualize the 5 things you feel grateful for. Notice how you feel and think. Every detail. Notice your breathing.

Now notice all the emotions you feel. Notice the positive messages of their presence.

"You belong. You bring joy and laughter. You are appreciated. You are fun to be around. You have a good life and much to be grateful for."

Repeat 3x.

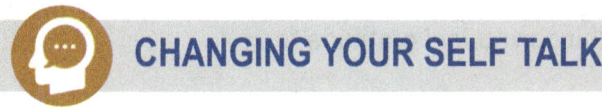

CHANGING YOUR SELF TALK

I change the way I feel with a smile. There are at least 5 people who bring a smile to my face. There are at least 5 times I can recall smiling and laughing. There are at least 5 things I am grateful for.

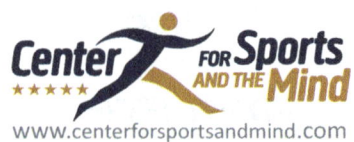

www.centerforsportsandmind.com

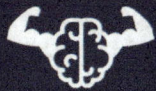 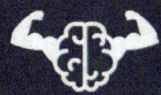
47. Mental Skill – Focus

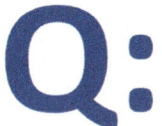 Where do you put your focus?

On things you can't do or can't control? On things you can do or can control?

Where you put your focus is where you put your energy.

Try the following exercise.

For the next 60 seconds see how many things you can count in the room that are blue.

Then close your eyes – ask yourself how many things you noticed that were white. You can't do it because that's not where your focus was. It is the opportunity cost of focusing on blue. Not noticing the white is the cost of focusing on the blue.

Many times, in sports we believe punishment is the best and only teacher. A focus on punishment may mean you miss important details and nuance that will help you improve.

What part of your inner athlete do you focus on most? What does that focus make you neglect? Does that focus help you avoid or confront something difficult or something you feel you cannot solve? Where does your focus need to shift?

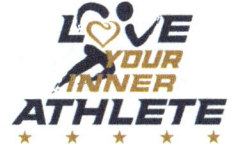

Do the following focus exercise.

Step 1 – Identify 3 objects that stand out around you.

Step 2 – Identify 3 colors that stand out around you.

Step 3 – Identify 3 sounds that stand out around you.

Step 4 – Identify 3 smells that stand out around you.

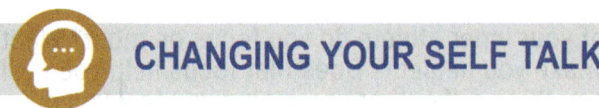

CHANGING YOUR SELF TALK

I direct my focus to what I can control. I focus on what I can do. I focus on ways I can use my strengths to improve my growth areas. I focus on my ability to learn and change.

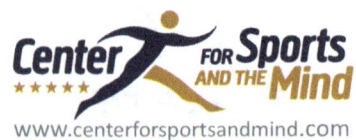

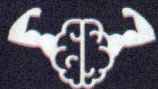 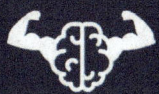
48. Mental Skill – The Injury

Q: What's the worst injury you have had?

What's the worst injury you have witnessed?

Serious injuries often bring up strong feelings because you care about your teammates.

Many times, injuries affect our ability to focus on the now. We may drift to worries about our teammate and lose track of performance.

We may get overwhelmed by anger or think the game does not matter. Both are normal reactions but don't help you or change reality.

You can recover a performance focus with a few quick and effective steps. These steps are listed on the other side of this card.

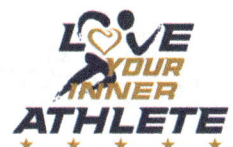

Follow the Injury Recovery Stretch (IRS) to help when recovering from injury. Start by stretching a muscle you can easily stretch.

Step 1 – Move your eyes left to right (they can be open or closed). Do this for the entire exercise.

Step 2 – Now pay attention to the muscle you are stretching. As you stretch, focus on your breathing. Inhale with the stretch, and then slowly exhale.

Step 3 – Hold the stretch for 20 seconds. Repeat the process again with the same muscle group.

Step 4 – When done, practice tensing and relaxing all your muscles until you have progressed through all parts of your body.

Step 5 – Give yourself permission to compete and turn care of teammates to those qualified.

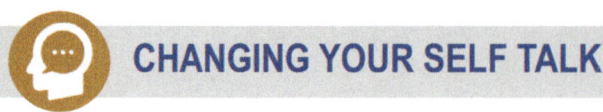

CHANGING YOUR SELF TALK

I use the IRS to mentally recover from injuries of myself and teammates. I give myself permission to compete after an injury to a teammate. I accept that overcoming injuries is part of the game.

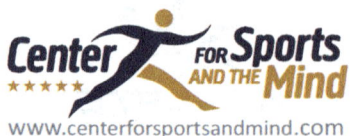

Center FOR Sports AND THE Mind
★★★★★
www.centerforsportsandmind.com

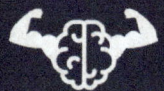 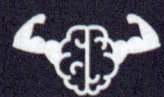
49. Tomorrow – Procrastination

Q: How often do you say, "I'll do that tomorrow?"

Do you follow through?

Procrastination often appears as a solution. We put things off because we don't feel ready, so we try to get out of it. Avoiding rarely does more than make it worse. It confirms how terrible it will be. Its negative power grows. Then it happens. There is no more time left. Action is required.

You need to answer for it: you are out of shape, tired, and unprepared. Someone is mad at you, or you have created a highly tense and pressured situation. You then think "why didn't I just do it?" or "if I had taken more time, I would have done so much better."

There is the pay off for procrastinating. An excuse for failing.

You can change this pattern. Attack the difficult things as the first task of the day. This approach works as you don't carry dread all day and build the belief that you can complete the most uncomfortable tasks.

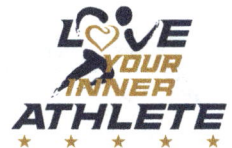

Don't wait or hesitate do this self calming exercise.

Step 1 – Locate the spot right below your armpit along your ribcage.

Step 2 – Tap 15 times. Without moving your head continue to tap and look up and to the right, then to the left. Then make a circle both clockwise and counterclockwise.

Step 3 – Repeat 5 times.

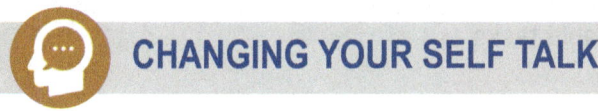

CHANGING YOUR SELF TALK

Procrastinating makes tasks more difficult. I am proactive with difficult situations. I feel better all day when I do the hard things first. I prevent drama by being proactive.

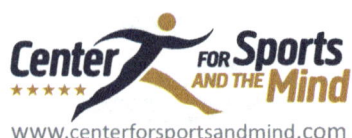

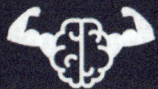 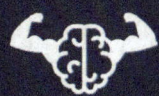
50. Who Do You Want To Be?

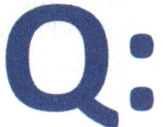

Are you being who you want to be?

Its one of the most important questions you can ask yourself. How do you know?

The process of being who you want starts with your values.

What do you value? What's important to you? Why is it important?

Step 1 – Write down 4 values that are important to you. Identify at least 4 reasons they are important to you.

Step 2 – Ask yourself the following questions.

1) Am I playing and living in a way that fits with my values?

2) Am I playing and living in way that respects the game, myself, and my opponents?

3) Am I playing and living in a way that builds self–trust, and trust in the process of development?

4) Am I giving my best effort in training, play, and prep?

5) Am I open to learning from the game?

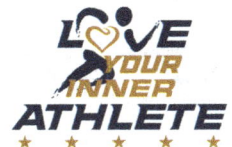

After reflecting on who you want to be, do the following exercise.

Get a 6-foot string and put 3 beads on it of different colors or 3 different colored marks on it. Put the first bead out 4 inches, the next 15 inches, and the next 30 inches. Tie one end to a doorknob. On your voice recorder app, record yourself calling out each color. Alternate colors. Avoid using a predictable pattern.

Record for 3 minutes. Move your eyes to the bead called out. You should see an "X" when you look down the string. Watch it move as you move your eyes. Repeat 2 times.

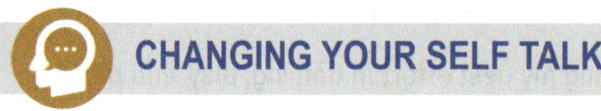

CHANGING YOUR SELF TALK

I play and live in ways that show my values. I respect and honor the game. I build trust in myself and my teammates. I trust the process to develop my game. I work hard and believe effort creates excellence. I know I develop when I learn from the game.

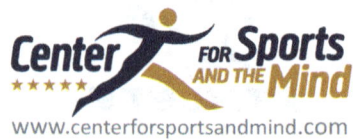

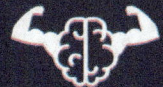 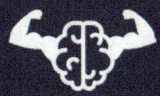
51. Your Ego – Your Opponent

Q: Are you the toughest opponent you have faced?

How often do you beat yourself up? Sometimes we are our own worst enemy. Why? Our egos get in the way.

Its job is to protect us from the criticism and uncertainty of performance. It also protects us from great performances.

Would you rather fail yourself or have the world fail you? This question summarizes the ego problem.

Some athletes chose the 1st option. When you make that choice, your performance will be tentative. You will play to avoid losing. You fear embarrassment and its vulnerability. You are in a Catch 22. There is no avoiding risk. No safe play. Damned if you do, damned if you don't. Playing all out or tentatively leaves you vulnerable to be embarrassed.

The solution – play all out. It is more painful to fail with regrets than to fail with none.

Sitting out is the only safe play but may be the most painful. It's not an option if you want to maximize your performance.

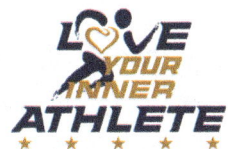

After letting go of your ego, do the following breathing exercise.

Step 1 – Begin by breathing in through your nose and out through your mouth. Imagine breathing through the soles of your feet.

Step 2 – Visualize your breath slowly moving up your body. Muscle by muscle. Relaxing your body as it moves up.

Step 3 – Visualize your ego. Create an image of what it looks like.

Step 4 – Have a conversation with your ego about the Catch 22. Let it know you are going to play all out and are willing to risk vulnerability.

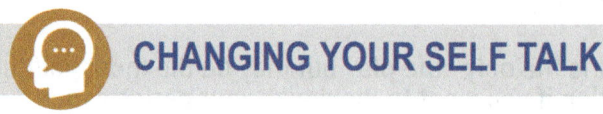

CHANGING YOUR SELF TALK

I play all out. I accept that I cannot protect my ego. My belief in myself is strong and I don't use my ego to protect it. I accept that vulnerability is a part of performing. I want to compete and not sit on the sidelines.

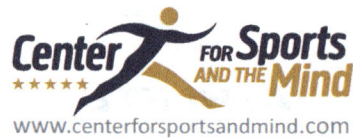

www.centerforsportsandmind.com

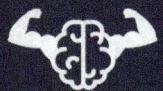 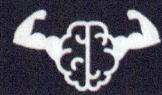
52. Constant Judgment

Q: Do you still like me?

Ever been asked this question?

If asked once, its OK. If asked repeatedly it is annoying at best and relationship killing at worst.

Athletes often get stuck in a loop of asking themselves that question. It is known as constant judgment. With every play, you judge yourself. You look at your performance in simple terms.

Consistent athletes suspend judgment and view their performance through multiple lenses. Getting stuck in the loop of constant judgment leads to overthinking, tension, and pressured performance. You are not playing in your OPZ. When checking a minute-by-minute score card, you don't focus on the task at hand.

It gets you stuck in the past and jumping into the future.

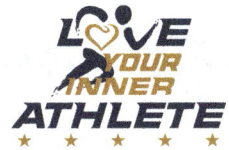

After thinking about those experiences go through the following steps.

Step 1 – Visualize your breath relaxing your core and moving down your body. All the way to your toes and up to your head.

Step 2 – Let your breath and relaxation help you identify judgments that interfere with your performance.

Step 3 – Imagine a power greater than you removing your judgment.

Step 4 – Watch the weight of the judgment leave your body and the feeling of lightness and relief that results.

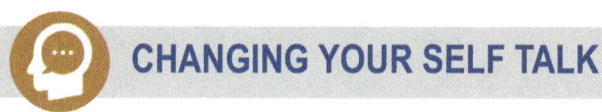

CHANGING YOUR SELF TALK

I suspend judgment and just play. I practice patience when tempted to constantly judge my performance. I use my resources to correct fundamentals. I accept that there is no one answer or solution. I trust my self and ability to change my performance.

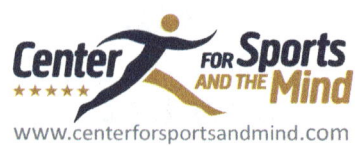

www.centerforsportsandmind.com

REFERENCES

1. Sinek, Simon (2009, September). How Great Leaders Inspire Action. Retrieved from https://www.ted.com

2. Childre, D. L., Martin, H., & Beech, D. (2000). The HeartMath Solution. San Francisco, CA: Harper SanFrancisco.

3. Grand, D., & Goldberg, A. S. (2011). This is Your Brain on Sports: Beating Blocks, Slumps and Performance Anxiety for Good! Indianapolis, IN: Dog Ear Publishing.

4. Shapiro, F. (2001). Eye Movement Desensitization and Reprocessing (EMDR): Basic Principles, Protocols, and Procedures. New York: Guilford Press.

5. Shapiro, F., & Forrest, M. S. (2016). EMDR: The Breakthrough Therapy for Overcoming Anxiety,

6. Dweck, C. S. (2017). Mindset. London: Robinson.

7. Duhigg, C. (2013). The Power of Habit: Why We Do What We Do and How to Change. London: Random House.

8. Farhi, D., & Young, B. (1997). The Breathing Book: Good Health and Vitality Through Essential Breath Work. East Roseville, N.S.W.: Simon & Schuster.

9. McGonigal, K. (2017). The Upside of Stress: Why Stress Is Good for You, and How to Get Good at It. S.l.: Avery.

10, Covey, S. R. (1996). The Seven Habits of Highly Effective People: Facilitator guide. Provo, UT: Covey Leadership Center.

11. Cabane, O. F. (2013). The Charisma Myth: How Anyone Can Master the Art and Science of Personal Magnetism. New York: Portfolio/Penguin.

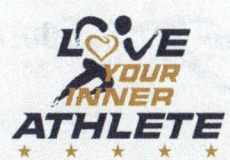

REFERENCES

12. Peters, M. A. (2012). See to Play: The Eyes of Elite Athletes. Minneapolis, MN: Bascom Hill Pub. Group.

13. Davis, K. (n.d.). How to Manage Worry. Retrieved from https://www.kathydavis.com/how-to-manage- worry/

14. Luber, M. (2009). Eye Movement Desensitization and Reprocessing (EMDR) Scripted Protocols: Basics and Special Situations. New York: Springer Pub.

15. Sincero, J. (2018). You are a Badass at Making Money: Master the Mindset ofWealth. New York: Penguin Books, Penguin Random House LLC.S

16. Hadfield, C. (2014, March). What I Learned From Going Blind in Space. Retrieved from https://www.ted.com/talks/chris_hadfield_what_i_learned_from_going_blind_in_space

17. Hallowell, E. M., & Ratey, J. J. (2017). Delivered from distraction: Getting the most out of life with attention deficit disorder. New York: Ballantine Book

18. Callahan, R., & Trubo, R. (2013). Tapping the Healer Within: Using Thought Field Therapy to Conquer Your Fears, Anxieties and Emotional Distress. London: Piatkus.

19. Foster, S., & Lendl, J. (2001). Peak performance EMDR: Adapting Trauma Treatment to Positive Psychology Outcomes and Self Actualization. Portale Italiano de Psicotraumatologia e Psciopteri

20. Hickman, L., & Hutchins, R. (2010). Eyegames: Easy and Fun Visual Exercises, an Occupational Therapist and Optometrist Offer Activities to Improve Vision. Arlington, TX: Sensory World.

21. Maley, M. (n.d.). Bioenergetic Fundamentals. Retrieved from https://www.scribd.com/document/76664165/B ioenergetic-Fundamentals Stress, and Trauma. New York: Basic Books.

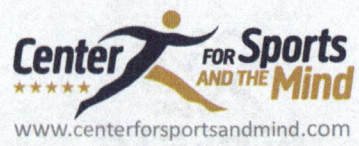

www.centerforsportsandmind.com

Made in the USA
Monee, IL
01 July 2024

60876969R00066